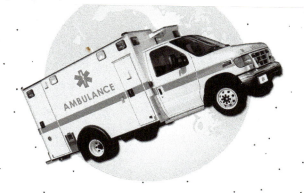

CALL NIGHTS

"Just don't hurt anybody!"

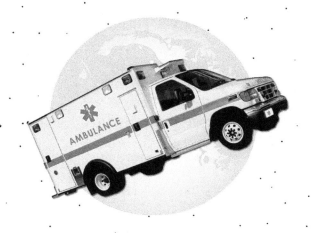

CALL NIGHTS

"Just don't hurt anybody!"

Kyle Smith

DO, PhD, FACP

Adriel Publishing

Forney, Texas

CALL NIGHTS

© 2012 by Kyle Smith

Published by
Adriel Publishing
709 Mulberry Ave.
Forney, Texas 75126

All rights reserved

FIRST EDITION

ALL RIGHTS RESERVED. No part of this book may be reproduced in any form whatsoever, by photography or xerography or by any other means, by broadcast or transmission, by translation into any kind of language, not by recording or otherwise, without permission in writing from the publisher, except by a reviewer, who may quote brief passages in critical articles or reviews.

Printed in the U.S.A.

Cover design by Brian Moreland & Liz Lawless
Interior design by Brian Moreland
red phone © Jose Manuel Gelpi - Fotolia.com
ambulance © Robert Wilson - Fotolia.com
stars © morrbyte - Fotolia.com
moon © losw - Fotolia.com

ISBN-10: 1892324024

ISBN-13: 978-1-892324-02-3

www.dockylesmith.com

Dedication

For...being my brothers, being there for me when I had no one...
you may not have chosen me, but I chose you...
William S. Howard, M.D.
George R. Welch
M. Keith Lewis
Jay Glen Westmoreland

For... teaching me how to take care of people, the RIGHT way...
Karl R. Brinker, M.D., C.M., F.A.C.P., F.R.C.P. (C)
Dallas Nephrology Associates

For...all you have given me...
Dana R. Smith

Contents

Preface: Call Nights	*ix*
Part One: Internship and Residency	**1**
1. The First Call Night	3
2. Learning the Ropes	21
3. How to Make it Through a Call Night	37
4. Dr. Heart—Code Blue	47
5. Night Rounds—Roof Call	55
6. Trysts	65
Part Two: Fellowship	**77**
7. Fellowship Call Nights	79
8. Shit Tickets	93
Part Three: Private Practice	**103**
9. Trolls	105
10. Some People Just Can't Take Care of Themselves	117
11. Code Me!	127
12. Become a Legend—Make a House Call	137
13. The Good Samaritan	147
14. Waxing Philosophic—On Call Nights	155

15. On Arrogance—On Call Nights	165
16. The Curbside Consultation	173
17. The Fair	181
Part Four: The Mentor	**189**
18. Worst Call Night Ever	191
Afterword	205
About the Author	211

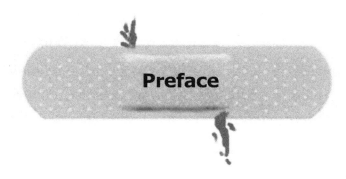

Preface

There are things about most occupations that workers either simply tolerate or detest altogether. I guess it depends upon the extent to which one gets annoyed with certain aspects of his occupation as to whether or not he gets to the point of telling the boss to take this job and . . . well, you know what I mean. Still, most of us tolerate those parts of the job, for me, outside of pelvic exams, *I hate call nights!*

Call nights represent the largest intrusion into my life I could ever experience. And, as you will see, it's not just because people get sick at night and we are charged with taking care of them. No, sir—there's something strange that occurs in the minds of people when the sun goes down. It is almost as if the common-sense neural pathway requires sunlight, or it becomes totally nonfunctional. Some of the things nurses and patients do at night absolutely defy logic, and, of course, it ALL must be reported to the on-call physician. Sometimes I stay awake after these calls wondering to myself, "Did I really hear what I think I just heard? Did the nurse just say that? Did the patient really do that?"

We get introduced to call nights as third-year medical students—and at that point in your medical career, it is way cool. It's even *fun!* You get to stay up all night, carry a beeper, discuss various things related to life and medicine with the nurses, and act as if you know what you are doing as a doctor. At that time of night, only the most seasoned of nurses can really tell the difference. It's the first glimpse a medical student has into the real world of being a doctor, and we think it is *the best*.

Then along comes internship, and some of the fun goes out of it as we realize we really don't know nearly as much as we thought we knew, constantly fielding relentless calls from nurses wanting to "just make you aware." Pretty soon you're ready to choke the ever-loving shit out of the next person who calls to tell you a patient has fallen out of bed … "just to make you aware."

When residency arrives, we've had a year to become

smarter about handling the majority of the real crap you get called about *and*, now we get interns to take the majority of the "scut"—the most boring, mundane, and demeaning work ever found in medicine. During residency, the young doctor starts to relish sleep time, so the classic statement to the intern goes something like this: "Call me if you need me. But remember, to call is a sign of weakness." That usually does the trick. Many needless calls are thus diverted from the resident on call, now taken by the hapless intern. The intern soon realizes why he or she is called "the wedge." The wedge is the simplest tool known to mankind, functioning solely to keep a door propped open.

Fellowship call nights start to approach real-life private medical practice. No resident or intern wants to deal with a night call for a patient with some form of chronic disease about which the *fellow* is honing his skills. That kind of call provides the perfect "dump," putting the call off on someone else, feigning ignorance. Fellows are smart enough to learn their way around this cat-and-mouse game to some degree, and ultimately, as I learned during my days working as a plumber's helper, shit really does run downhill. Being in the valley, the wedge will be up to his or her ass in, well, let's just say one will have a lot of mundane things to do in fairly short order.

One would think that as the doctor enters private practice, the night-call fun would be replaced by real-life emergency calls from the sick, injured and dying, or from those who must care for patients during a "deep night" shift. That is where you would be wrong; in fact, it gets worse, and in most circumstances, the beloved wedge is not there to help. The the realization hits: YOU are now the wedge again. It strangely resembles a circle-of-life kind of thing.

The following text is a collection of real-life stories and calls I've had to field, along with some of the drama associated with each of these stories. These include incidences from internship, residency, fellowship, private practice—and definitely some weekend call stories. Hearing these stories for the first time, I am sure you'll be as amazed as I was while looking back, shaking my head, and wondering if these people will ever pull their heads out of their asses. I do have my doubts—and know for a fact that some of these people *never have*. Some stories are sad, as happens in real life and, you'll read my views on them. Maybe you will agree and maybe not. But the beauty of the human race is that we are all different, yet alike in so many ways. What we think can be wrong, but how we *feel* can never be wrong.

The book is divided into four parts: internship/residency, fellowship, private practice … and the fourth, as you'll see, a very special part to me. After each story is a section called "post hoc," from the Latin phrase meaning "after this". These are my reflections on the significance of each section in terms of learning about life, medicine, or myself. The "post hocs" were created well after these stories were originally written. When necessary, I have used fictitious names. I hope you enjoy these stories—and I would write more, but I'm on call tonight. Damn, *I hate call nights.*

Part One
Internship and Residency

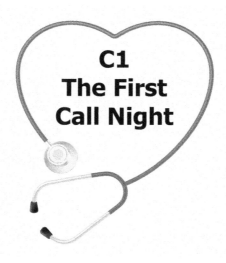

C1
The First Call Night

For me, there was no greater feeling than graduating from medical school. I felt as if I had just conquered the world and knew everything there was to know about everything in medicine … and I FINALLY got to be called "Doctor." I was really looking forward to internship and residency, getting to put into practice all that I had learned, or thought I had learned. The incoming intern class at the hospital where I trained attended an orientation for three days prior to July 1, the day all internships and residencies commence. We were treated like kings and queens, each with an orientation package with his or her name on it, of course preceded by "Dr."

At the end of the orientation, we were given two lab

coats with our names embroidered on them—with "Dr." in front of our names, of course—and issued our pagers. Our very own pagers, the kind that talk to you, the ultimate gift, a rite of passage, and something that signified one's importance. Little did I know that soon I would want to cram that damn pager up the ass of the very next person who called and squawked, "Dr. Smith, please call …"

When July 1st came, I was giddy with anticipation. I was assigned to the internal medicine ward service for my first rotation, and I was on call the first night of internship. I was ecstatic; nothing could be better. I spent the first day traveling the wards with my resident, Billy, as he explained the rules and hierarchy of the residency. He also gave me a crash course on the different floors, the "nuances" of the various nurses, and showed me the ICUs, which seemed to have all the very pretty, young nurses. When five o'clock rolled around, the nightly ritual occurred. All the call residents and interns changed into scrubs, donned lab coats, and ate dinner in the cafeteria to ready ourselves for the long night ahead.

I think Billy could tell I was a bit nervous from the first night of being an RD (Real Doctor). He told me, "Hey, man, I'm here if you need me. Try to do what you can by yourself. But if there's something you just can't figure out or just flat out do not have a clue, ***do us both a favor—don't hurt any-***

body ... just give me a call. I'll be in the call room catching a nap. If the ER calls you for a hit, just go down, get a look at it, and then give me a call. We'll decide what to do with it and I'll come down and help you, OK? Don't worry, you'll do fine."

"Thanks," I replied. "I appreciate it. And I'll try not to bother you."

I went into the call room and broke out *Harrison's Principles of Internal Medicine.* All of a sudden I realized, I really didn't know as much as I thought I knew. I got this rather sick feeling when the first call came: "Dr. Smith, please call 3 Central."

Oh, shit.

I knew, from Billy's orientation, that it was the nephrology floor—kidney patients, the sickest of the sick. And transplant patients. I knew jack shit about transplant medicine. "Damn," I thought, "why didn't I just do psychiatry or research and be a rat doc." I put it off as long as I could; then I called.

"This is Dr. Smith, someone paged."

"Are you the intern on call?" the nurse asked.

"Yes, I am."

"Good, Dr. Schwartz forgot to write TPN (total parenteral nutrition) orders for Mr. Cash. He wants you to come write them for him."

"Uh, OK ... I'll be up in a minute."

"We need them written pretty quickly; the pharmacy is already bitching. They have to formulate it right away."

"OK, sure. I'll be right there, as soon as I take care of what I' m working on."

Of course, I was "working" only on trying to settle myself down and remember something from medical school that might actually help me. I quickly turned to the *Harrison's* chapter on TPN. It was far too long to read, and I couldn't quickly assimilate anything that would be remotely helpful to me. So I went on up to 3 Central to scope things out.

"Are you Dr. Smith?"

I answered with a quick and nervous, "Yeah."

"Well, here's Mr. Cash's chart; the TPN orders are in the front. Dr. Schwartz just told me to tell you to prescribe the same thing as was written for yesterday." Whew! I was relieved—I had never written TPN orders before. I didn't know half the crap they put in that stuff, let alone trying to prescribe it for someone. So I filled out the form, signed my name, and went back to my "intern on call" room.

Before I got back there, the pager went off again. "Dr. Smith, please call 5 Northwest." Shit. Oncology.

I stopped at a hall phone and called. A patient had passed

away, and they needed me to come and pronounce him dead. I found a very old man, wasted away from age and prostate cancer. He was 92. I listened to his chest for a heartbeat, and felt for a pulse—both absent. I went to the nurse's station and asked for the patient's chart. I quickly found the name of the attending physician and looked at the progress notes. The patient had been moribund for a few days, given medications to keep comfortable. The last progress note said, simply, "Patient comfortable. Death is near." I wrote a death note in the progress notes section, documenting my exam in detail, and finished up with a brief sentence: "Patient pronounced at 2315. Attending notified."

The attending physician was Dr. Stephanie Welch, a brilliant hematologist/oncologist, but a mean and nasty woman if you crossed her—all this courtesy of Billy's briefing earlier in the day. I asked the charge nurse if she could put a call in to Dr. Welch so that I could tell her of her patient's death. The nurse, Angie (what a bitch; I'll have more to say about her later), asked, "Are you sure?" which I thought was rather strange.

I replied, "Sure, I think she needs to know her patient passed away."

Dr. Welch promptly returned the call. Angie said, "Dr. Welch, please hold the line for Dr. Smith." She transferred it to me.

"Hello? Dr. Welch, this is Dr. Smith. I just wanted to notify you about the passing of Mr. Benson. I just pronounced him."

Her response, "What the hell time is it?"

She had obviously been in a very deep sleep, as her voice was deep and slow.

"It's about 11:30," I answered.

"And you are who?"

"I am Dr. Smith."

She cleared her throat. "Well, DOCTOR Smith, what is your first name? Because I know it's not doctor."

"Uh, Kyle, Dr. Welch …"

"OK, *Kyle,* I want you to listen really closely, OK? I am a cancer doctor. I have patients die every day. I know they are going to die. I write it in my notes, if you bothered to look. And I don't mean for this to sound like it's going to sound, but I really think you need to hear it now, being so new to this profession: DON'T EVER FUCKING CALL ME IN THE MIDDLE OF THE NIGHT TO TELL ME ONE OF MY PATIENTS DIED WHEN I HAVE WRITTEN ALL OVER THE CHART THEY ARE TERMINAL AND I EXPECT THEM TO DIE ANY MINUTE! You got that? Did I make myself clear?"

Quivering, I responded, "Yes ma'am. You made that perfectly clear, and I assure you it will not happen again."

"Good, Kyle, make sure it doesn't."

Click. She hung up.

I sat there for a minute, stunned. Angie said with a smirk, "I asked you if you were sure you wanted me to call her ... and you said yes."

About that time the emergency room started to page me about admissions. Between midnight and 3 a.m., I got hit with nine admissions. I called my resident down to help me, and he zipped through those admissions like he had been doing them all his life.

"So, how's your first night so far?" he asked.

"Well, I'm kind of reeling from nine hits in three hours, and I got to meet Dr. Welch tonight on the phone. She's a real sweetheart."

"You didn't call her about a dead patient, did you?"

"Yeah, I did. I thought you were supposed to call the attending when a patient died. I didn't know."

Billy just laughed. "Man, I'm sorry. I should've told you. What a fucking bitch. Don't worry, in the next three years you'll get it again. She just needs a man—till then, she'll add your scrotum and balls to all the others she has hanging on her wall. It happens to all of us. Let that shit roll off your back. Hey, it's time for me to go crash. You think you can bed down the last two?"

"Yeah, I can do that."

"OK. Be sure to wake me up for morning report. You have to present all these cases to Dr. B (the internal medicine program director). Call me at 6:30, OK?"

"Yeah, OK."

As I was finishing my last patient and hoping I could get a couple of hours of sleep, that pager went off again. "Dr. Smith, please call 3 Central."

I called them back. "This is Dr. Smith."

"Are you the intern on call?"

I subdued the overwhelming desire to scream, "Of course I am, you fucking moron. Why the hell else would I be calling?"

Instead, I answered with a simple, "Yes."

"We've had a patient fall out of bed, and you need to come check them."

I quickly learned that, truly, all of the shit runs downhill in the hospital, and the lowest life-form is the intern, residing firmly in the deepest valley. And *every* patient who falls out of bed must have the intern check him out. I told 3 Central I would be up as soon as I could.

When I arrived, they pointed me to the room of a very

young patient who had just received a kidney transplant. She was getting out of bed to go the bathroom and tripped. The room was dark when I went in, so I turned on the lights. The floor nurse accompanied me. I introduced myself to the patient and told her I needed to check her out. She was very nice. "OK," she said, "but I think I'm just fine, and I really want to get some sleep."

"Well, this won't take long. I just need to do a really brief neurological exam to make sure everything is OK."

I completed the quick mental-status exam and peripheral exam, then examined her head and then asked for the lights to be turned out so I could check the response of her pupils to light and dark. I shined the light into her eyes; they were the clearest eyes I had ever seen and so green. But the pupils did not respond to light. I just couldn't figure out what was wrong.

The patient asked, "What are you doing?"

"I'm trying to check your eyes."

"I don't have any eyes. Those are prosthetics."

The nurse quickly said, "She's blind."

I felt like crawling into a hole. I just said, "Oh . . . hey, I'm sorry about that. Those are still very pretty, though." I mean, what can you say to cover up what a dumb ass you are?

I knew word would spread like wildfire about that little

incident, and I was right. Never lived that down, for three years.

Just when I thought that first night had mercifully ended, another call from the ER came in. A woman had been found face-down on a river bank, halfway in the river and halfway out. The police were called because someone thought it was a dead body. But when the police rolled her over, she opened her eyes, and she was brought posthaste to the ER. She was dehydrated and had been lying in a bed of fire ants, and was caked head to toe with river mud.

I called Billy back in; he was none too pleased. After we examined her and wrote admission orders, he said, "Let's take her down to physical therapy, put her in a Hubbard tank, and clean this old gal up. She smells like a rotten oyster." So we took a nurse with us, filled the Hubbard tank with iodine soap and water, and proceeded to scrub the mud off. I asked Billy if he thought we should do a pelvic exam, in case she has been raped and left for dead.

He was clearly frustrated by my suggestion. "OK," he said reluctantly. "I don't want any part of that. Go ahead and run your hand up her crotch if you want."

I gloved and tried to do a vaginal exam, but quickly realized that no one could have raped her; her vagina was packed with mud and gravel. When I told Billy, I thought he was going to spit his Coke everywhere.

"That's just beautiful. Nice work. Can't wait for Dr. B to hear this one."

I had barely enough time to grab a cup of coffee and head in for morning report. I presented all of the cases to everyone assembled. Dr. B filled out an index card on every patient and kept them in a little gray box. When I presented the case of the woman found in the mud, I left out the vaginal-exam portion.

But Billy was not about to let me get out of that one. When I finished stating my physical exam findings of the heart, lungs, abdomen, and skin with all the ant bites, I went on to present the lab.

"Excuse me, Dr. Smith," Billy interrupted. "You DID leave out another portion of the physical exam."

"Go ahead, boy, tell me what you left out," said Dr. B.

I told him about finding the mud and gravel in the vagina. He *did* spit coffee out, then chuckled a bit and said, "OK, let's name this one Gravel Gertie. And next time you're curious about something like that, get a gynecological consultation for your patient. Sounds to me like you need to leave that for the pros."

I handed that damned call beeper off to the intern replacing me as quickly as I could. What had started out as a beautiful night of being a doctor, *finally,* had ended as an embarrassing debacle of just how much of a dumb ass I really was. I had been chewed out by a mean attending, failed to recognize a blind person, and admitted the now-famous Gravel Gertie along with the other nine admissions. I had to work another 12 hours the next day. I couldn't wait to get home and crash.

This was the introduction to call nights for me. Little did I know what was to come.

Post Hoc

The process of becoming a doctor is much more than a four-year journey through medical school. It is truly a lifetime adventure. There are so many things about medicine and taking care of people that can never be taught in medical school; it constitutes only a mere introduction to what is to come.

Graduating from medical school is a tremendous accomplishment, but it also comes with tremendous responsibility. As hard as medical educators try to convey that fact to their students, it doesn't really hit home—until that one case comes along. It's the one that requires everything a young doctor can conjure up from medical knowledge and common sense to save that person.

The pitfalls are legion. One of my favorite movies from years ago was *Gross Anatomy*. The one thing I always remember from that movie is what the anatomy professor tells the entering class and writes on the chalkboard the first day: "Alcoholism, drug addiction, suicide, divorce."

"Congratulations," the teacher tells the class. "You just took your first step into a profession where these things are more prevalent than in the general population." It is very true, and I never understood why until I was in practice for many years.

The internship year is very important, yet I believe the intern should come away from that year being proficient in only two things:

1) Knowing how to take care of the patient. That is, writing orders nurses can understand, caring for the patient day to day, documenting that in the chart, and finally, making appropriate deposition.

2) Learning to recognize what IS sick and what IS NOT sick. Now, this is the difficult part—it may sound like a simple undertaking, but I can assure you, it is not. There are many brilliant doctors in practice, filled with book knowledge, who have never been able to master that one thing. It takes much more than book knowledge to become a good doctor.

If the intern can come away with these two skills in the

first year, that internship has been a success. The rest of residency is where pure diagnostic and procedural skills should be honed.

I'll always remember that first night and the sheer terror of that first call asking me to write TPN orders. "What did I learn in medical school?" I thought. At that particular moment, I remember thinking I hadn't learned *anything*. Of course, that wasn't true. I did know something—just not what I thought I knew.

The progression that must occur in the new physician's mind during the internship year is best described as a curve, plotting time with months across the bottom of the graph and medical knowledge along the side. What typically happens with the curve is the following: Month one sees medical knowledge at a perceived high. The successive months, toward month six, sees a *decline* in that curve as the new doctor's confidence of what he or she knows waivers and ultimately reaches a nadir. The last portion of the internship year sees a progressive rise in the curve, back toward near the starting point, but it never reaches where the intern thought he was at the beginning. For some, that drop in confidence occurs in month one. For me, it occurred on DAY one.

William S. Howard, M.D., was my resident. We struck an instant friendship that lasts till this day. I don't know what it was about Billy that made us instant buddies, but I do know that I could not have gotten through my internship or even the better part of my life without him. We have seen each other through some great times and some very difficult times. He is the godfather of my son, and I am godfather to his daughter. He has had his practice and life business to attend to and, God knows, I have had my own to deal with. We don't talk or see each other as much anymore; life will do that to you sometimes. But I do know that, just as on that first night on call, I could call him anytime and he would be there for me, as I would for him. He is a phenomenal doctor and the best friend anyone could ever have. I never had a biological brother...and though he might not appreciate it, except when the bar tab comes my way, I chose him. I love him very much.

Armand G. Schwartz, M.D., is a gastroenterologist who was attending physician during my training. He is one of the brightest and best gastroenterologists I have ever had the pleasure of working with, and he is an absolute wizard with an endoscope. He is in there and out *in a hurry.* He and I became friends and played more than a few rounds of golf together during those years. Armand, if I ever have to have something shoved up my ass, you are my guy!

Stephanie Welch, M.D. (not her real name), could truly

be a real bitch in every sense of the word. She had a very low tolerance for people who were not as smart as she was—which included most everyone. Hematology/oncology was never really my thing. I had two rotations with Dr. Welch during my residency. The first time, I couldn't sleep the night before because I knew she was going to fucking rip me a new asshole.

But she turned out to be an amazing teacher, and I gained a true respect for her skills as a physician. And while the entire house staff was fearful of her, her patients absolutely loved her. She was a hard woman, in that she never minced words with any of her patients or colleagues. Dr. Welch never sugar coated anything, and I heard her say some very direct things to patients. Yet she had compassion that you could see only when she interacted with patients. I learned a great deal about communicating with patients as I watched her. By the time I was a senior resident, she trusted me to take care of her patients for her and, while I am still not entirely certain, I think we *almost* became friends. In later years when I became an ER attending, we had a great professional relationship.

Cancer is a terrible disease, and it takes way too many lives way too early. And while I pray to God, if he listens to me anymore, that I never get that disease, if I do I would be most glad if Dr. Welch took care of me.

Jack Barnett, M.D., M.A.C.P. —Dr. B—was an unbelievable character from Bovina, in deep West Texas. Legend has it that there was a time when he was considered by many the best diagnostician ever, and a complete wizard at the bedside, striking an instant rapport with patients. Right out of the country, he used to say that it was only for pure etiquette that a surgeon would politely knock the cow shit off his boots before going into the operating room, because it didn't really matter what was below the sterile field.

He once posted an article in the residents' conference room titled, "Who is the Poor Historian?" ... a perfect reflection of his philosophy and person as a physician: *Listen* to the patient, and if you do it long enough, he will tell you what is wrong. I looked at Dr. B as a father figure, certainly not perfect by any stretch of the imagination, hardened by life and medicine, but tempered by the years and everything that life and medicine taught him. I will forever be indebted to him. Dr. Barnett recently passed away; it made me very sad. One of my colleagues went to visit him a few days before he died. He said that even on his deathbed Dr. B was still full of piss and vinegar. The interesting thing is that he still tried to teach and impart some wisdom to my colleague. I hope his soul gets some rest.

The lessons and the scars of that first night and first year stay with me always, and I think, because they do, I have been a better doctor.

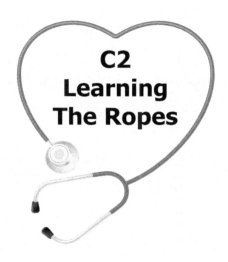

C2
Learning The Ropes

Taking night call is part of being a doctor—the unsexy part. It doesn't take a new doctor long to figure that out if he or she is smart at all. And if you are a slow learner, you have every third or fourth night to try and figure it out. The other thing you figure out as an intern is that nurses love to call you, for pretty much everything. You are their private physician, available to them twenty-four hours a day, someone they can call when they have questions, to harass when they have nothing better to do, and to provide never-ending fodder for their gossip. I have always believed, but never been able to prove, that each nurse randomly picks her own special intern, and then it becomes her special project to absolutely demoralize and completely make that person's life a living hell. I was one of the lucky ones; I had *three* nurses who "picked" me: Carrie in the coronary-care unit, Angie (I told you I would have more to say about her) on 5 Northwest, the oncology floor, and Tara in the ER.

Carrie was a very young nurse just discharged from the Army. I often wondered if it was honorable, dishonorable, or if she was told to leave and simply reported AWOL, marked DNFFBD (Do Not Find, Fucking Brain Dead). She always worked deep nights; 11 p.m. till 7 a.m., and had the specific knack of always looking busy, but never really accomplishing anything useful. She was soft-spoken, careful to enunciate everything properly, and could give you a presentation of a patient that in no way, shape, or form related to anything going on with that patient. The only thing you could trust about what she said was the patient's name and where to find them…and sometimes she got *that* wrong.

One night, in the midst of multiple hits (admissions) from the ER, I received a page: "Dr. Smith, please call CCU." I knew who it was before I even called.

"This is Dr. Smith, someone paged me."

"Yes, Dr. Smith, this is Carrie and I have a question about Mr. Hilton. Are you familiar with him?"

This was then, and is now, a pet peeve of mine. I want to

scream at the top of my lungs every time I hear that question. "Have you seen my fucking name on the chart anywhere? Then that must mean I am NOT familiar!" I know this kind of question is just medical foreplay, but it still pisses me off.

"No, Carrie, I'm not. What's your question?"

"Well, Mr. Hilton is a seventy-two-year-old white male with COPD (chronic obstructive pulmonary disease) and pneumonia. He was admitted yesterday by Dr. Garner, and he seems kind of anxious, not able to sleep, and I was wondering if you could just order some Ativan or something to help him rest."

Well, there were a few things about this little conversation that really bothered me, in addition to the "Are you familiar?" question. First of all, Dr. Patricia Garner was an overly aggressive pulmonologist, or lung specialist, noted for eviscerating interns and residents when they made stupid mistakes. Secondly, if Mr. Hilton had been admitted to the CCU, that meant he was really sick and maybe close to being placed on a ventilator, perhaps needing to be intubated (a breathing tube placed directly into the lungs) and mechanically ventilated. Finally, when a lung patient is anxious, it may be simple nervousness—or it could be that they are getting sicker. Because I was so busy, I almost made the classic intern mistake: simply ordering what Carrie wanted. But having had a "history" with Carrie on call nights, I opted not to.

"Carrie, what are Mr. Hilton's vital signs?"

"Wait a minute." she answered. I heard her put the phone down and walk to retrieve her nursing notes and flow sheet. "OK, let's see, his temperature is 100.5 degrees Fahrenheit, his pulse rare is 100 and irregular, and his blood pressure is 130/80."

The one piece of data I wanted, she failed to give. "Carrie, what are his respirations?"

She didn't answer for a second or two, and then said, "Yes sir, he is."

"Is WHAT, Carrie?"

"He is respiring. Breathing. Isn't that what you wanted to know?"

I shook my head. "Carrie, how many *times a minute* is he breathing?"

"Wait a minute." She put the phone down again, and I heard the pitter-patter of nursing feet scurrying off into the distance, and exactly one minute later, I heard that pitter-patter returning to the phone.

"OK. Dr. Smith? Are you there?"

"Yes. Carrie, just tell me the respiratory rate."

"OK, Mr. Hilton, the seventy-two-year-old COPD patient of Dr. … "

"Carrie, SHUT THE HELL UP. I ALREADY HEARD THAT PART. JUST GIVE ME THE FUCKING RESPIRATORY RATE!"

"Sorry, Dr. Smith. It is 42 times per minute."

The normal respiratory rate is somewhere around 10 to 16 breaths per minute, depending on how pissed off you happen to be at the time.

"Carrie! Get a respiratory therapist there stat, draw an arterial blood gas, move the crash cart in there, and I'm on my way."

Cool Al, the anesthesia intern, heard this diatribe, and as I was getting ready to bolt out of the ER, he asked, "Hey, man, what's up? You need some help?"

"Carrie," I said, "is trying to get me to murder one of Garner's patients. He's crashing. Come running if you hear the code pager go off."

Cool Al just shook his head. As I ran off, I heard him say, "That bitch ain't got sense enough to pour piss out of a boot."

When I arrived in the CCU, Mr. Hilton was in severe respiratory distress. I asked for the crash cart to be opened.

"Do you want me to push the code button?" the CCU charge nurse asked. "Not yet." I wanted to ask whether it was for the patient or for me!

I asked her to put a Miller blade on a laryngoscope and to retrieve an 8.0 French endotracheal tube (which is inserted directly into the lungs) from the crash cart. The respiratory therapist returned with blood-gas report, which confirmed my suspicion. Mr. Hilton was "anxious" because he was grasping to find any molecule of oxygen available to him. He was in acute respiratory failure, and would code in a matter of seconds if I did not intubate (the act of placing a breathing tube into the patient) and ventilate him. To have given him something for his "anxiety" to calm him would have given him the sleep of his life, something I call a "dirt nap." I would have knocked out *all* of his respirations and killed him.

I quickly intubated him, put him on the ventilator, and stabilized him. I called Dr. Garner and let her know what had happened and that the patient was now on the ventilator. "Good work, Smith," she said. "Now get a repeat ABG in an hour and have them call that to me. We'll talk about the physiology of hypoxemia later this morning, OK?"

"Yes ma'am, Dr. Garner." I didn't have the balls to tell her that Carrie had tried to set me up, and that I had almost killed her patient.

The second of my appreciation club, Angie, was an "older" nurse. I really can't tell you how old, but when I was an intern, she seemed damn near ancient and still wore the old-style nursing cap I had previously seen only in pictures. She also worked deep nights on the oncology floor. There was no other nurse in the whole hospital who loved calling the house officer on call more than Angie. She would call me to come see a patient and after I left the floor, she would wait just long enough—she had it perfectly timed and knew when I was just getting into the call room—and then she would call again.

One night when I was on call, Angie almost single-handedly caused me to turn in my scrubs, throw the pager into the shitter, and tell her to grind everything into a medicinal powder and just blow it out of her ass. At 11 p.m., she called me to evaluate a patient who felt short of breath. I ordered an electrocardiogram, an arterial blood gas, and a chest X-ray. I evaluated the patient, found nothing more than a little wheezing—which he had upon admission—and ordered breathing treatments every four hours. She asked me if I would see another patient who was feeling anxious while I was up there. I complied, and ordered a Xanax for that person. All of this took about an hour and a half. I started back to the call room and *as soon as I walked in* and saw that inviting bed, I heard, "Dr. Smith, please call 5 Northwest."

"Dammit! I was JUST up there," I thought. I called while looking at my unmade bed with its nice clean sheets. "This is

Dr. Smith. I was just up there."

Angie answered: "Yes, I know, but after you left Mrs. Fowler in 5040 said she couldn't sleep and wanted a sleeping pill."

"Fine. Give her Restoril, 15 milligrams now and repeat it in two to three hours if it is not effective."

I went to the restroom to take a leak and *finally* I was ready to hit that nice warm bed. But when I sat down to take my shoes off, there it went again. "Dr. Smith, please call 5 Northwest."

I was about ready to come unglued. I called immediately and SHE answered. "5 Northwest, this is Angie." If I could have grabbed her throat through the phone, I would have. "This is Dr. Smith, what do you want now?"

I could hear giggles in the background. "Well, Mrs. Marsh in 5015 is having some chest pain." By now I had my head in my hand.

"OK, get an electrocardiogram stat. I'll be back up there."

I stormed back up to the fifth floor. When I arrived, the EKG had been done and was normal. Not only that, Mrs. Marsh was fast asleep and snoring like a rhino. I was so pissed I could hardly see straight; then I decided to inflict a little payback. "Oh Angie, could you get me the charts of the patients I have seen for the past three hours?"

She did. I wrote further orders on each chart. Since it was 3 a.m., I figured I could get another two sets of vital signs on each patient before change of shift. The nurses *hate* vital signs because that means they must obtain a blood pressure, heart rate, respiratory rate, and temperature. Nowadays they generally have nurses' aides to do this task—funny, *doctors* don't have that kind of help. Usually the vitals are taken once a shift, but since I *did* make therapeutic interventions, I reasoned that it wasn't unreasonable to track those interventions. So I wrote orders on each of the patients I had seen, for Angie to take vital signs every two hours till 7 a.m. I placed the charts with the orders in a neat stack at the nurse's station.

"Anything for me to do?" Angie asked with a grin.

"As a matter of fact, yeah," I answered. "Good night." I walked down the hall toward the elevator with a big grin on *my* face. Then all of the sudden I heard, "Dr. Smith, wait a minute. You want vital signs every two hours on these patients?"

I never once turned around and looked at her as I continued toward the stairs. I just called back, "Yes ma'am, I do. Wait a minute, you only need to do Mrs. Marsh once, since I didn't really make a therapeutic intervention on her. And I'll be back at 7 a.m. to look at those vitals. Thanks so much for your help."

I took a quick look back. Angie looked as if she had been hit by a truck: mouth wide open, and that old nurse's cap now sitting sideways on her head. Needless to say, she wrote me up for that one, and I had to have a little visit with Dr. B, my program director. He laughed, slapped my hand, and told me to behave ... but it was worth every minute of it.

The third charmer on my rounds was a veteran ER nurse name Terri, she was tough as an old work steer. Interestingly, she and I became quite good friends in subsequent years, when I was an attending in the ER after my training. If someone was truly sick, she was Cracker Jack. But if they were faking it, or she thought they were faking it, she could be your worse nightmare. She exposed the patients she thought were full of shit via the way she wrote the complaints by the names of those patients. That was back in the days when you actually wrote the names of the patients on a large ER board next to the room numbers, so that everyone could see who was where and what their problems happened to be. Designators such as "abdominal pain," "chest pain," GSW (gunshot wound), or "vaginal bleeding" were written under the CC (chief complaint) column.

Terri's favorite complaints to write about those patients

she couldn't stand were NVPOS (Nonviable Piece of Shit) and TOBASH (Take Out Back and Shoot in Head). She also had a lust for trauma and hated "medicine patients." She loathed having to take care of them but was occasionally forced to do so when the hospital was filled and a patient was waiting on a bed. She was and is a very good nurse; she takes really good care of the sick. I love her dearly to this day.

One night I was just getting hammered with admissions. This was back in the day, before there were limits on the number of hits or the number of hours one could work in a day. I had admitted this little old man with chronic kidney failure, who was due to initiate dialysis. Terri was complaining about how she had to take care of this "renal troll." By the time I had finished everything, it was 3:45 a.m., and I just wanted to get a little sleep. I made it to the call room and fell asleep straight away. At 4:45 a.m., the pager went off: "Dr. Smith, please call the ER." After a sentence full of expletives, I called and got Terri on the phone.

"Hey, Smith, this old renal troll down here says he hasn't taken a shit in about a week. You didn't write a laxative for him."

I guess Terri had compassion for the sick old man. Wait a minute ... no she didn't, she just wanted to wake me up. It pissed me off so much that I told her, "Yeah, OK. Well you can give him 30ccs of 70 percent Sorbitol by mouth. BUT you can't give it till 6:30 in the morning, when normal people get up to take a shit!"

She answered, "Have you lost your fucking mind, intern?"

"Maybe I have. But don't ever call me again for a laxative at 4:45 in the morning."

Well, I probably shouldn't have said that because she went right to Dr. B about it. I think I amused him, because he laughed his ass off when I told him the story. But then he quickly added, "You know you gotta stop doin' that shit, don't ya', boy? I don't want to see you back up here again gettin' in no pissing contests with these nurses. Just because they don't treat you with respect doesn't mean you have to treat them the same way. Besides, trust me—with that nurse, you ain't gonna win that one."

While learning the ropes of call nights, a very important lesson was imparted to me: Nurses can be your best friends, or they can be your worst enemies. And when it comes to trying to keep some element of sanity or get any sleep at all, you need all the friends you can get.

Post Hoc

I don't know whatever happened to Carrie (not her real name). I suspect she ultimately became a damn good nurse. She was very young, and I think I was a little harder on her than I should have been, but she just frustrated me so much. Still, I needed to take the high road, and I didn't. I'll always feel somewhat badly that I never told her I was sorry for berating her, both in front of her face and behind her back. Yet another thing I am certain God will punish me for.

Cool Al—Alan Raphael, M.D.—was a great guy to hang out with on call nights. He was very bright, somewhat quiet, and had a really dry sense of humor. He made me laugh my ass off a number of times. I know he loved sleeping people, and he remains a top anesthesiologist today. In fact, he is one of the few I could trust to "sleep me," but more important, to wake me up. As Cool Al taught me, it takes nothing to put them down; the trick is bringing them back.

Dr. Patricia Garner (not her real name) recently passed away. I was very sad to hear about that. Her career was cut short by a bevy of neurological issues, many of which I never understood completely, although rumor had it that she treated herself with large doses of steroids. She was very aggressive, both with her patients and with the interns. No matter how you wrote an order, she *always* changed it. For example, if you wrote for Lasix 40mgs IV; she would change it to Lasix 40 mgs twice a day by mouth, and vice versa. The residents had a euphemism for when you got a lecture from her: You had been "Garnerized" or had "Garneromas" all over you. Deep down, you could tell she was a lonely woman—never married, and I seriously doubt she ever dated. I mean, who in their right mind would put up with her shit? Still, I always got along well with her, regardless of the etiology of her problems and her intimacy issues.

I felt sorry for her when she told me about all this heavy lifting she had to do around her house, so one Saturday, I helped her haul some shit out of her garage. She gave me two filing cabinets full of landmark medical literature and articles she had saved, about every disease known to man. I think all the residents think we had an "intimate encounter"; I know I took a lot of shit over it. I hope they believed me when I denied it and told them all to go fuck themselves. With her passing, I think medicine lost a very good doctor.

Angie (that may have been her real name, I don't know) was just a pure bitch, and stupid. And, believe me, that is no way to go through life in medicine. She has most likely long since retired, or may have passed away. She almost single-handedly killed one of Billy's clinic patients, a ninety-seven-year-old nursing-home patient. I have a whole handful of stories about mistakes and medication misadventures directly related to Angie that I had to deal with over the three-year residency. Suffice it to say, some people just should not take care of other people, regardless of how much they think they want to.

Terri (not her real name) was and is one of the best nurses I ever worked with—smart, very smart. A confident single lady her whole life, she met an accountant and they had a quick romance that didn't last; I think she probably screwed the poor guy into submission...and good for her for doing it. Unfortunately, Terri found out why he was over 50 and had never been married: Momma wouldn't let him. And I thought there was a cutoff age for sleeping with your parents. Luckily, she met another man. They married and, to the best of my knowledge, remain happily married in Colorado. I wish her the best; God knows she deserves it.

Now I know one thing that is *critical* to learn in those early years is how to deal with nurses. They can be best your very best friends and keep you out of a lot of trouble, or they can be your worst enemies and nightmares. The best advice is this: Treat them all well, and learn those you can trust and those you cannot.

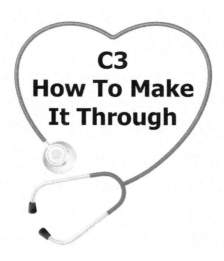

C3
How To Make It Through

Part of the requisite training of a young doctor includes learning little tricks of the trade to negotiate call nights successfully. Learning these tricks constitute the ultimate on-the-job training; everyone picks up their own little secrets along the way. These tidbits are primarily designed to give the on-call nurse something useful to do—because an idle nurse equals frequent calls. The more you can give the nurse to do, the more time you'll have for the precious commodity of sleep.

The first thing one must learn to make it through a night on call is that no matter how busy you are, *always stop to eat.* I learned this from one of my upper-level residents,

Richard Baker, M.D. He required that no one do any work at all between 5 and 6 p.m., and we could all be found during that hour in the hospital café and grill. The trick was to stuff yourself, because you might not get another chance to stop all night. I have seen several variations on how to accomplish this. Some people would get their food to go, head back to the call room, and eat lying down, thus killing two birds with one stone. Savvy residents would always take a little extra and hide it in the resident call room refrigerator, hoping to retrieve it later. Another nice trick was to stuff your lab coat with candy, gum, and mints; it only takes an extra meal ticket, and those little items can calm even the meanest of the nurses.

The next trick was learning how to be stealthy; a resident who is not seen is one less resident to grab curbside for a quick scut-work job. There are various ways to do this, but I preferred using stairwells and surgical corridors that were vacant during the evening hours. I even discovered some passages long since forgotten—or not passed on to future resident classes. And one should *never* walk the halls just for the sake of walking the halls; no, sir—that is an open invitation for being granted some unpleasant task.

A trick that takes years to hone is the one of taking a call about a particular issue, and having ready in your armamentarium a carefully thought-out plan that will afford the maximum amount of sleep time. These plans need to be based on solid medical literature and an acceptable way to handle a particular problem, but also designed to keep the nurses busy. Here are a few of my favorites.

A predictable call would come in about 11:30 p.m. most nights, right after the evening vital signs were taken. Blood pressures out of the ordinary were always reported to the on-call doctor. In the majority of circumstances, the blood pressure would be modestly high; the patient would have received his or her nighttime blood-pressure medication dose about 10 p.m.; and it would not have yet had time be absorbed from the stomach and to reach therapeutic levels. The trick starts with explaining to the nurse and telling her to recheck the blood pressure in two to three hours—depending upon how much sleep you need. This would mean the next call would come about 2:30 a.m.

Now, here's the real trick: There was a landmark study written a number of years ago out of University of Texas-Southwestern Medical School and Parkland Memorial Hospital Dallas, which advocated a way gently to lower the blood pressure with medication by mouth every one to two hours. *Perfect, and generally effective!* At 2:30 a.m., the nurse is told to take the blood pressure again in one hour; if the blood pressure is above whatever parameters one sets, the nurse on duty should give 0.1 milligrams of Clonidine by mouth, wait one-and-a-half hours and repeat the blood pressure again. If it remains above the parameters, the order may be repeated another two times. That's another four-and-a-half hours, and gets you from the 2:30 a.m. call all the way to 8 a.m., when the attending or the other ward team can deal with it.

The sleeping-pill calls have always driven me nuts. I mean, how much sense does that make? If you haven't fallen asleep by 3 a.m., why worry about it? Not only that, but now you've woken me up and we *both* can't sleep. I think they should put a copy of *Harrison's Principles of Internal Medicine* in every room; just open that up and start reading—it's guaranteed sleepy time within three pages. I especially used to hate the calls explaining that the first sleeping pill didn't work and asking for another, to which I would answer, "Sorry, NO. No Marilyn Monroe disasters on my watch."

Since so much of a sleeping pill is placebo anyway, in my opinion, the best formula I could devise was giving a low dose of a mild benzodiazepine, with the order that it could be repeated in two to three hours if needed, equaling a full dose. If the patient or the nurse was particularly demanding, I would give only an antihistamine, and if they were very nasty, they had to give it by injection in the ass.

The late night "Doctor, the patient seems disoriented" calls are particularly distressing. Those will generally require a visit, but there is a way to postpone it as long as possible. When getting one of those calls, it's essential to make sure there is nothing metabolic, infectious, or something to decrease the oxygen level in the bloodstream as the etiology. This is the cool part: You can check all of that with a bevy of lab work! Just order a CBC, a basic metabolic profile, and an ABG, or arterial blood gas, and you have a wealth of information. Plus, it takes three hours minimum, plenty of time for a catnap because if anything is grossly abnormal, it will be reported right away. Just tell the nurse to call you when it all comes back. This entire process works very well, provided the patient's vital signs are OK.

One can even use the nurses for nifty little wake-up calls if one is prone to sleeping through morning report. Just time the lab correctly, or leave an order to be notified of this or that at the appropriate time; works like a charm.

These are but a few of the tricks employed by the savvy house or staff officer to negotiate a night on call successfully. There are others, but some secrets are best left secret.

Post Hoc

Richard Baker, M.D. (not his real name) was an upper-level resident when I was an intern. He was always a bit strange, but incredibly brilliant. He trained at Harvard and subsequently did a fellowship under one of the country's most respected experts on hypertension. I was never really good friends with him; I don't think anyone was. He died a few years after the residency of complications from HIV. Too bad—a bright physician and years of training lost. I have often wondered what he would have accomplished.

I have learned over the years that a good working relationship with nurses is essential in taking good care of patients. They should always be treated with the utmost professional respect because not only are they educated professionals, but also they do a job that no one could pay me, or most doctors I know, to do, certainly not for what they get paid. I sometimes do not know how they do it, or why they do it.

Just as with doctors, there are good ones and bad ones, those whom you can trust and those you cannot. We all have horror stories about mistakes nurses have made, but I can share some egregious mistakes that *doctors* have made as well. In *every* circumstance, the doctor must assume responsibility for the care of his or her patient. That means if there's any question in your mind about what you're being told, you go and see the patient, day or night. There is no substitute for being there—you can defend almost anything you do if you are at the bedside, making the evaluation yourself and carrying out a treatment plan. This is something a few doctors have never really learned, but ultimately will ... the hard way.

The other side of the story is that some really sharp nurses can and have saved the asses of many interns and residents. You don't hear these stories because rarely will a doctor admit that he didn't know what to do or that he just screwed up. But I am going to share a story with you about myself that I have told before to nurses, interns, and residents about how nurses can save your ass.

Tommy Hughes, R.N., was one of the very best nurses I ever had the pleasure of working with. A battle-hardened ER nurse, Tommy had seen *and* done just about everything. Later, Tommy became one of my most trusted ER nurses; he could be trusted because he knew what he was doing, and he could function independently. We also had a great relationship, and he was one of the reasons why I was able to stay as long as I did in the ER. On those long ER nights, Tommy and I shared some of the most hilarious stories. I would repeat them here, but I think some stories are best left alone.

Here's one I can tell, though. When I was an intern, I was called by Tommy to come see one of our patients from the internal-medicine clinic. The patient was very sick and while I was in the room, she lost her heartbeat and stopped breathing. Tommy immediately started chest compressions, called for a nurse and respiratory-therapy help, then looked at me and said, "Doctor, she's coding." I remember standing there, thinking "Shit! What the fuck do I do now?" I must have had that "Oh, shit!" look on my face, and Tommy recognized it. I had taken advanced cardiac life support before, and it didn't even register that I needed to implement it. Tommy immediately took control, but did it in such a fashion that was subtle and non-threatening.

"Doctor, you want us to go ahead and push the epinephrine while you intubate her?"

I snapped out of it. "Yeah. Go ahead."

The respiratory tech handed me a laryngoscope already assembled, and an appropriate-size endotracheal tube. Luckily, I got the patient intubated. About that time, Tommy asked, "Doctor, are you ready for 1 mg of Atropine now?"

"Yeah, go ahead."

"Doctor, do you want me to hold compressions now?" Tommy continued guiding me in his subtle way. "Do you think that is a good rhythm on the monitor now?"

I looked. The patient had a rhythm. I checked the pulse; she had one. And about that time, Tommy said, "Her blood pressure is 120/60. Good job, Doctor. You did good."

Yeah, right. Tommy saved the patient, and my ass. He knew it, and I knew it. As we were taking the patient to the ICU, it was just him and me in the elevator with the patient.

"Hey," I told him, "Thanks for saving my ass tonight."

"You did just fine." He smiled at me and patted me on the back. "You're gonna be real good."

Once I was an ER attending, Tommy and I told that story probably a hundred times over the several years I was there, and we got a good belly laugh each time we told it. Tommy is retired now; he tried to do massage therapy for a while. I don't talk with him anymore, but I love him like a brother to this day.

C4
Dr. Heart
Code Blue

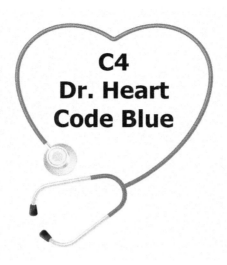

On call nights during residency, one is required to wear the "code" beeper. Each resident on call was required to carry one, and to respond to the unit or room where the code was called. In our hospital, rather than have the pagers scream, "Code Blue ICU!" they squealed "Dr. Heart, ICU!" I think this was because *everyone* knows what Code Blue means ... at least anyone who has watched *Ben Casey, Medical Center, Marcus Welby, M.D., General Hospital, St. Elsewhere, ER, Grey's Anatomy,* or *House.* And because I did my residency in a large hospital system, the damn code beeper went off all too frequently.

The worst-case scenario is having the code beeper fire

off when you have finally retired for the evening. A quick scramble out of bed, dead sprint toward the staircase, up the stairs two and three at a time, and the home stretch down the hall to the ICU, only to be paged again: "Cancel Dr. Heart. Cancel Dr. Heart." Well, by this time, your metabolism has received a quick bolus (large dose all at once) of epinephrine, norepinephrine, and a blast of steroids from your adrenal glands. Kind of hard to go back to sleep after that, but you learn. This type of "pseudo code" was usually perpetrated by some unsuspecting new nurse who, in the course of gossiping about hospital people, leaned against the code button, setting code beepers off in the middle of the night.

In genuine code situations, all of the interns and residents converged on the room, along with the primary nurse, the charge nurse, a couple of other voyeuristic nurses, the respiratory therapist, and the chaplain. Generally it was standing room only. As the resident gets savvier, once an appearance has been made, the situation assessed, and it's been determined that all the help needed is present and accounted for, a stealth exit can be executed in the back hallways to the call room for a blissful nap. Unless, of course, you happened to be the unlucky bastard who made it there first; then it was, by default, your show, and the other residents were able to execute *their* exits.

Early one morning about 1 a.m., the pager sounded, waking me out of a deep sleep and, likely, some erotic dream. "DR. HEART, 4 Northwest." Out of all the call rooms, you could hear a collective, "Shit!" As we all converged on the room on 4 Northwest, we found a little old man, lying at a thirty-degree angle and not breathing, with a nurse attempting to ventilate him with a bag and mask. I immediately asked those assembled to lay him flat, start chest compressions, and prepare to code and intubate him. But when they hit the button on the electric hospital bed to place the patient supine, his body stayed at its thirty-degree angle! The patient was already in rigor mortis, and his body was fixed in the position in which he died. I quickly placed one of my hands on his chest, the other on his leg, forcing his body into a position close to supine, so that we could actually code him.

I went through the motions, "buffing the chart" to make it look like we gave the old man every opportunity to be resuscitated, just in case a litigious family or an ambulance-chasing attorney caught wind of this. The entire exercise was like trying to resuscitate a cadaver. After I called the code and pronounced him OFFICIALLY dead, I asked to see the nurse's notes. The floor charge nurse retrieved them for me. This man had to have been dead for a few hours, yet the nursing documentation indicated normal vital signs at 11 p.m.

Not only that, but the nurse had also documented that the patient took a glass of water at 12:30 a.m.

The charge nurse asked me what I was looking for. I explained to her that the man was already in rigor mortis, and I thought he had passed away a few hours before. She refused to believe it, and called the primary nurse and asked her if her documentation was correct. The primary was adamant that it all happened just like she said. I just said, "OK. But I'll bet he really drooled a lot when you gave him that glass of water." I left it at that because the chart indicated that the old man was a chronic end-stage lung patient. He had obviously died, mercifully, in his sleep. It really was the very best exit he could have hoped for, except for having insult added to injury, as the little nurse tried to drown him, too.

Yet another early morning—this time at 5:30 a.m.—another blaring on the pager: "DR. HEART, ICU. DR. HEART, ICU!" After the usual expletives, I raced toward the ICU to find CPR in progress on a renal transplant patient. One of the "high power" renal fellows from "the best medical school in Texas" was making early rounds and was in attendance. Since he was the senior of the physicians present, he, by protocol, was the guy in charge—and was he acting the part, barking orders out here and there, watching the cardiac monitor intently, and screaming for drugs to be pushed. I think he had been watching a too few many of those doctor-type shows. This "M.D. thing" sure appeared to go to his head.

I stood back and watched the show, figuring that it was too late to grab any significant kind of nap. So I grabbed a Diet Dr Pepper and enjoyed what I thought was the most hilarious comedy I had seen in a while. This code took on a life of its own. The fellow just kept saying in a panicked voice, "The patient is still in coarse V-fib. Let's shock him again!" I thought this was a bit strange; I think the old son of a bitch had received enough electricity through his chest to light up New York City. I was afraid he was going to be fried to a crisp, with nothing left for the undertaker.

I had never seen anyone remain in ventricular fibrillation that long, so I positioned myself so that I could see the cardiac monitor. I took one look at this mysterious coarse ventricular fibrillation rhythm. It looked a little too symmetrical to me—more like artifact. I looked at the EKG leads from the defibrillator; they were hooked up correctly. As I followed the wires to the patient, I saw that they weren't *on* the patient; the leads were planted firmly in the floor. It was all I could do to keep from spitting Diet Dr Pepper all over the room. I held my tongue for a second, and then I figured I would have a little fun with the Nobel Prize winner from "the best medical school in Texas."

One of the really sweet little ICU nurses was enthralled with this whole scene. I tapped her on the shoulder and said, "Hey, watch this." I walked toward the bed past the fellow, bent down, and picked up the leads off the floor. Everyone was stunned, including the asshole fellow. I got close enough to his ear to say, in a very low voice—but one I think most could hear anyway—and said "Congratulations. You just successfully coded the floor. You might want to hook these up to the patient."

I turned around, took a drink of Diet Dr Pepper, winked at the nurse, and calmly walked out of the room. A couple of my resident friends were heard howling with laughter as they exited the room. The nephrology fellow didn't speak to me again for the rest of the year.

Post Hoc

Learning how to orchestrate a resuscitation attempt successfully is yet another task to be learned in the invaluable residency years. And it is important to take charge; the resuscitation team looks to one person to direct the show. I never understood why we all needed to respond to every code called at the hospital, but by the time my residency was over, I understood completely. The more you see and do, the more you learn, and the better you become at it.

I wish I had not made an issue of the code I ran when I found that the little old man had been dead for some time before the code was actually called. As old as I am now, and as long as I have been doing this kind of thing, if I had it to do over again, I probably would not have said anything. Just figuring that the little old man had died a quiet, serene death in his sleep, I would have talked with the nurse one-on-one. She would have probably denied it anyway, but I would, in a professional way, have simply let her know I knew.

The renal fellow got too excited to check the most basic thing prior to making any kind of therapeutic intervention—that is to make sure you know *what you are treating* before you treat it. Now, I understand how that can sometimes happen, and I know it is something that needs to be considered every time one has the urge to jump in and treat, but the doctor *must* ask himself, "What am I treating? If I don't really know, how will the treatment affect the patient if I am right or if I am wrong?"

Sometimes we must "shoot from the hip," but most of the time we are afforded time to make a logical determination.

The renal fellow in this story is a wonderful doctor, one of the best renal transplant physicians in the country. We have since become friends, and I see him occasionally at medical conferences across the country. He has never once mentioned the "floor code" incident to me. And I wish now that I had not embarrassed him as I did—but it was just too funny. And those opportunities just don't come along all that often. It still cracks me up.

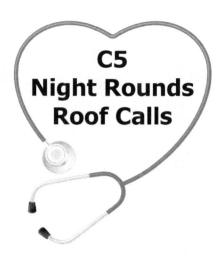

C5
Night Rounds
Roof Calls

As you go through residency, it's sometimes necessary to break the monotony of call nights. Most of the various techniques for doing this have been handed down from house staff for generations; others are simple variations of old tried-and-true techniques, and still others are brand new and specific to a particular house staff class. A couple of my personal favorites were old standbys.

The hospital where I trained brought in a class of new nurses, fresh out of nursing school. Nursing recruiters would go to the individual nursing schools across the country, talk with the graduating classes, and offer new nurses signing bonuses, moving allowances, and generous shift differentials for those wishing to start out working nights. And many of these new nurses found that the night-shift differential was too good to pass up. The majority of the new R.N.s were all too eager to meet the house staff, many in search of that elusive "M.D. meal ticket." Rather than a M.S.N. (master of sciences in nursing), they were looking for the M.R.S. degree, "Dr. and Mrs.," that is. The interns really believe that the nurses are interested in them—and now, that even makes me laugh, partly because I was an intern victim myself. By the time you're a resident, you've figured things out and know the game all too well, but it makes for some really good fun *and* quite a diversion from taking care of a nursing-home patient with a rip-roaring urinary-tract infection.

After things would quiet down early in the morning, before retiring for a quick nap, one ritual was to take a quick jaunt through the unit with the best-looking nurses. You would just stop by, make it look like you were checking out a patient, read a little bit of the chart, and ask some really intelligent patient-oriented questions of the hot little nurse taking care of that person. This provided a perfect segue into a friendly conversation and chitchat; nurses *love* to chitchat. You could get a pretty good feel for a particular nurse's interest level during this short repartee, and generally that information was imparted to all of the house staff. That way, you didn't waste any precious sleep time on one that had a boyfriend or frankly wasn't interested.

Another ritual, this one handed down to a mere chosen few, was the nightly summertime rite of taking calls from the hospital roof. Once upon a time, a curious resident (his name rhymes with Billy), who obviously had nothing better to do, had done a little exploring and found an abandoned office with windowed roof access. The office was in the older part of the hospital, located strategically above the old ICU. The really cool part was that it had a phone that was functional, as well as a few chairs. The roof provided a panoramic view of the city, and on warm spring or summer evenings, provided a little break from the insanity. In subsequent years, with a little modification, this area became like a mini-resort.

The first thing we did was to procure a phone-cord extension, easy enough. Next, I figured out that if you're going to have a resort, you must have lounge chairs. These were smuggled in on a Saturday afternoon after rounds, utilizing a large box marked as if it was filled with medical supplies—perfect. The next thing I thought you needed in a resort was access to cold beverages. Now this was a little trickier, but I formulated a plan after I completed a transplant-medicine rotation. I noticed that the organs, once harvested, were placed in ice chests marked "Human Organs" or "Human Tissue".

These were kept in the surgical pathology lab which was easily accessible through the operating-room area. I "borrowed" a couple of these for private use. It was easy to carry whatever you wanted in these things while in the hospital, because no one wanted to look and see what was inside—clever, huh? A variety of beverages was procured for our new resort, some stolen right from the residents' lounge refrigerator, others brought in on special occasions.

Rusty, a third-year resident during my training, would occasionally end up being on call the same nights as me. I loved hanging out with him. He knew his way around everything in that hospital, and he knew the scoop on everyone. In addition, I thought he was a very good doctor. Rusty was into Zen and karma, and I think he could read people pretty well. We used to hang out on the roof a lot when we were on call together. We came to be close fiends and shared a lot of secrets; I trusted him implicitly. Any time I had a problem or a question, Rusty was there, ready with the answer. We drank a lot of beer together after work in those days.

While enjoying ourselves one summer night on the rooftop when I was an upper-level resident, one of the interns was invited to join me. "Do you think we ought to be doing this?" he asked.

"Have you always been this chicken shit?" I replied. "I'll

bet you were the class monitor in grade school, the president of student council, and a member of the debate team in high school, a ΦBK in college, and the top of your medical-school graduating class, weren't you? Don't be such a pussy. Just shut the fuck up and finish your drink. Make like a real doctor, for Christ's sake. Besides, we are done for the day."

He answered. "I don't think I was ever the class monitor in grade school."

Enough said. For me, getting out on that roof on call nights just made me feel a little more human at a time when I was generally treated like something less than that.

The best time of the year on the roof was summer, especially the Fourth of July. If you liked fireworks, there was no better place to see them. And it was Rusty's favorite thing to do in early July. Because the hospital was in a central location, all the firework shows across the city were in plain view. To get to see those, when you were stuck in that hellhole like a prisoner under house arrest, made you feel a little better and more normal . . . at least, it did for me.

Sometimes, when the group of residents and interns who were on call with you were really cool, we would all agree to "go out to eat"…not in the literal sense, however. Typically, really good pizza or barbecue would be shipped in.

All of these things helped maintain my sanity during

those resident and call-night years. Of course, that was many years ago. Today, you probably couldn't get away with half the shit we did. Nowadays they give the house staff days off, put a limit on the number of admissions they can accept in an evening, and restrict the number of hours they work in a week. I guess all that's another product of the "ME" generation. I like the way it was in the old days; I think we learned a lot of medicine, and we took really good care of people—just maybe not such good care of ourselves. But we had each other, and a lot of the time that was enough.

I was laughing with a very prominent physician friend of mine the other day. We trained together during those years. "You know," he said, "I really miss those nights up on that roof sometimes. The only thing we had to worry about was running out of food or drink, and getting caught. Seems like so little to have to worry about compared to being a real doc in these times."

"Yeah, I certainly do understand what you mean," I answered. "Hey, let's meet at that new rooftop bar in town. It won't be quite the same, but what the hell."

"I'll see you there in an hour."

Once there, we sat and talked about the old days as we looked out across the city once again. It was like being on call together once more, and we agreed to meet there again as soon as we could.

The hospital tore down that old building, toppling the resort we built from scratch with our own hands ... but all of the memories remain. And call nights have just never been the same.

Post Hoc

I sincerely believe that being in the position to take care of patients as they come in—as you are on call nights—mimics what private-practice medicine really is all about. Being on call overnight or over the weekend means you must take care of anyone and everyone admitted to your service. Going through intern and residency call nights prepared me for private practice in a way nothing else could have. Today, restrictions are placed on the house staff, such that after a certain number of hours worked or past a certain number of admissions, you get days off and have relief from more admissions. I frankly don't agree with this. I understand the logic behind these new standards: the powers-that-be are concerned about sleep deprivation and quality of patient care.

But in the real world, while sleep deprivation can and does cause one to be less sharp, it also requires one to concentrate—at least that's what it did to most of us who trained "back in the day". And you always had someone to help. I also believe the more you see, the more medicine you learn. I know there are many people who disagree … and frankly, I couldn't give a shit. I'm just that hardheaded. Anyway that's my opinion.

I look back on some of these call nights now and I realize they were the best call nights of my life, even though I didn't think so then. I learned that the call nights during internship and residency serve a purpose; they are invaluable in teaching new doctors medicine on a basic level. They teach young doctors to make decisions based on deductive reasoning and gut instinct. I still learn a great deal of medicine when I am on call, but that aspect of it has lessened through the years.

Russell Anderson Jones, M.D., remained one of my dear friends after our training. He took a position in a multi-specialty group about 60 miles or so from where we trained together. When Rusty entered into private practice, I would routinely make the hour-long drive down to hang with him. He always had the knack of making me feel better—better about myself, better about a particular situation, or simply better about life in general. Rusty was really good that way. We used to vacation with one another during our residency, and together with Billy, we had some absolutely incredible times together at the beach. We were like family; I never had any biological brothers, but back in the day, Billy and Rusty were as close as it comes without being blood-related.

A few years ago, Billy called me one afternoon. I knew immediately something was very wrong. His voice was slow and deliberate, and I could tell from his tone that he was very sad. "I have some really bad news," he said.

"What?"

"Rusty was just killed in a car wreck."

I was stunned. I don't even remember what either of us said after that. Rusty was apparently driving the family minivan into town; he lost control of the car and hit a bridge pillar. He was killed instantly. Billy and I went to Memphis for his graveside funeral service, but I still don't think the full impact of his loss hit me until years later.

There are certain things you are never prepared for … even when you're a cynical old son of a bitch like me. I think about Rusty often. I think of all the things I did not say to him that I wish I had. I don't know if Rusty was in the least bit religious; we never talked about it. But wherever his soul resides, I hope he is at peace.

I would be remiss if I didn't mention a couple of other people who helped me get through those nights on call, and I think I helped them too. In addition to Billy Howard and Rusty Jones, I have to acknowledge my very good friends,

Ronald K. Garcia, M.D., and Louis A. "Bud" Torres, M.D., they were like brothers, too. Our favorite thing was "Boy's Night Out". We had some fun times during those residency years. Both are successful internal medicine specialists today and remain dear to my heart. We shared a lot during those years, both personally and professionally.

I could call any of these guys today if I was in trouble, and I know they would be there to help. And I would do the same for them.

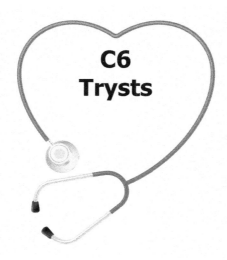

C6 Trysts

I have often wondered about the attraction nurses have to doctors. It is a multifaceted attraction, and one not always based upon looks, I can assure you. I think there is an inherent respect that nurses have for doctors—perhaps that is taught in nursing school or perhaps it is an acquired respect. I also think that things happen between people when you work so closely together; you develop bonds, working in concert toward a favorable outcome for the patient. Undoubtedly, there are also those circumstances when physical attraction plays a strong role. I think many nurses and other women, for that matter, see being a spouse or significant other to a physician as a worthy goal for secondary gain. And

I suppose I do have to throw in the possible scenario of two people simply meeting, falling in love, and getting married ... kind of like we were all told it should be. Wait a minute. That can't be right, can it?

Since the nurses were pretty much our age, all of us naturally hung out together, generally most every night. We had a lot of favorite watering holes back then, places such as Dick's Last Resort, the Outback Pub, the Ice House, and, in the summertime, usually some nurse babe's apartment-complex pool, replete with all the beer we wanted, courtesy of her refrigerator. It really is amazing how much better nurses looked in bathing suits as opposed to scrub clothes, but I digress.

Hollywood has certainly glamorized the personal interplay among doctors and nurses. Look at how many soap operas, bent on capturing the imagination of jilted housewives, are centered on themes of hospital politics, relationships, gossip, and the hot affairs of doctors and nurses. Hell, one of them is even called *General Hospital*. Truth be told, while glamorized somewhat, it kind of *really is that way*, at least to a degree. Even in the largest hospital setting, don't ever think for one minute that everyone in that hospital doesn't know everything about what is going on, all the way from the cleaning lady to the chief of staff. You can bet your sweet ass on that one. The really funny thing about it is that when one of these torrid affairs happens, the two people who are trying to hide it think no one knows what's going on. But in reality, EVERYONE knows. And when a doctor and a nurse are getting in a little extracurricular activity, it's so funny to watch their interaction with one another in a professional setting: little winks, funny little remarks, maybe a quick touch to the arm or shoulder. Too funny. Sometimes you want to just go up to them and say, "Hey, are you guys having sex? Because that is what everyone's been talking about!" But decorum prevents you and, realistically why would you take away some good cheap entertainment?

The critical error is to launch into one of these relationships and think that the nurse won't tell, at least, her closest nurse buddy. And then it's only a matter of time before it's all over the hospital. Remember, *nurses love to chitchat.*

And, of course, these little trysts are not restricted to just nurses and the house staff; even some of the most seasoned attending physicians have fallen victim to that trap. I will never forget a critical-care specialist who was head-over-heels for a quiet, pretty young nurse, recently divorced. He was married, but quite the playboy type: originally from England, blown-back haircut, dressed to the nines, an incessant flirt on rounds, and driver of a black Porsche 911. Ordinarily, when something went wrong with a patient, the nurse would call the resident on call to assess the situation. Depending on who the attending physician was, the resident generally took care of the problem, unless there was a question. In which case, you called the attending, he or she told you what to do, you wrote the orders, and the attending went back to sleep.

With regard to this couple, I first noticed over time that whenever she was on duty, Sloane always took care of Dr. Edward Walker's patients. I became suspicious that something was going on between the two of them when it was publicized, through the residents, that Dr. Walker wanted to be called on all of his patients at night, which struck me as a bit odd. My suspicions were all but confirmed one call night when I was asked by Sloane to come see a patient. "Dr. Walker asked you to come evaluate my patient and then call him back," she said. "OK, I'll be right there."

When I got there, the patient was in some respiratory distress. I didn't have time to call Walker back, so I just intubated the patient, got a chest X-ray and an arterial blood gas, and then I called him back.

I went over everything I had done, and he said "Perfect. You did a really fantastic job. I'll be right over."

"Dr. Walker, really, if you want to sleep, I think the patient is pretty stable now and I'll call you if anything changes."

"You're the best resident I have there, and I know you're

right, but I think I better come in to make sure on this one."

I went back to bed, and about an hour later was called back to the ICU to see another patient. I checked on Walker's patient. Sloane was gone, so I asked if Dr. Walker had been there, and was told he had. I asked where Sloane was, and someone said she was "on break." When I left the ICU, I saw her coming back from the professional building with that "tousled sex look" ... and then noticed Walker scrambling towards his Porsche, obviously hoping no one had seen him. The affair was confirmed later because Sloane did what every other nurse does, she told another nurse, and then it was everywhere.

I was on my apartment balcony one evening having a beer when I heard a little bit of noise coming from a unit just a couple of doors down from me. One of the ICU nurses lived there. The noise sounded, curiously, like the throes of passion. I sipped my beer and listened intently. After the blessed moment occurred—and it was easy to tell—I heard someone open the front door. I peered over my balcony to see one of the most prominent surgeons in the city, Laurence Williams, M.D., making a fast exit. He glanced up at me, then kept his head down and walked all the more quickly. He had clearly recognized me. I saw him a couple of day later in the hospital. He came up and talked to me like I was his long lost brother.

"Hey, I hear you hunt sometimes," he said. "How about a deer hunt on my ranch next month on a weekend you're off?"

"Sure," I answered.

Nothing was ever mentioned about the sighting, but I got a great hunting trip out of it.

There were many trysts among the house staff and the nurses, but, unlike Hollywood's portrayal, they really don't occur in broom closets. I *never* had sex with a nurse in a broom closet; I got mad, passionate kisses from a social worker in there one time, but we didn't have sex. Sometimes the little rendezvous happened on call nights. When they did, usually one of the residents would "Tom Sawyer" you into holding his beeper for a little while and tell you not to knock on the call-room door. Then they'd sneak the hot little babe ready for some fun up the back stairwell and enter the resident's quarters from the back way ... no pun intended. Sometimes the nurses who were off work would go have a few drinks, set up a meeting in the back stairwell, and come on up for some late night fun. Hell, some of them even had their own keys.

We were doing happy hour most every day with the nurses. Everyone knew that this person would be leaving with that person, and many times you could get a rundown of everything they were doing. Man, do nurses talk.

Yes, I am human. Yes, I have been morally tested. And yes, I have failed. I, too, fell victim to one of the prettiest, sweetest little nurses you ever saw. We had multiple little chitchats on call nights, and I really liked her a lot. But I wanted to maintain professional decorum and I didn't want to fall victim to the gossip bug I had seen run rampant so many times. Not to mention the fact that I thought there was no way in hell she would ever be interested in me. The house staff and the nurses frequently went to parties together, sometimes really good ones.

At one such get-together, Chris was there with some of her nursing friends and I had been there most of the afternoon. I saw her, said a quick hello, and moved toward the keg of cold beer. The house was packed and the bathrooms were filled. I needed to go take a leak and, being from the poor part of town, I naturally went outside to take care of my business. I stood there, enjoying my buzz, enjoying the pee, and enjoying the cool night. I finished my business, put everything back in its place, and turned around to go back into the house. Chris was standing right behind me.

Startled, I said, "Hey, I'm so sorry; I didn't know you were out here."

She didn't say anything; she just grabbed me and kissed me passionately. Then she said, "I'm sorry. I had to do that. I had to see what it was like." She laid another one on me and sighed heavily. "I know we can't do this. Everyone will talk. I know I shouldn't do this. I want to go home with you, but I can't. I'm so sorry." She turned and ran back into the house.

It took me a few days to process all of what had happened. Another call night rolled around, and I was called to the ICU to see one of her patients. We didn't talk; I just took care of the patient, documented everything, and wrote a couple of orders.

Chris finally came over to me. "Are there any orders for me?"

"Yeah, just a couple," I replied. "Hey, I just wanted to apologize for the other night. You know, you get a little beer in you, and you get out, let loose, and stuff like that happens. I'm really sorry. I hope it doesn't do anything to our friendship or working relationship."

"Well," she said in a very low voice, "I'm not sorry it happened at all." She slid me a piece of paper. "Call me anytime you want to talk or want to come over and have a beer." I was stunned. I called her the next afternoon and was over there within thirty minutes after work.

At parties and happy hours, Chris and I had an elaborate

little communication system. Her purse on the table meant she would leave first, and I would have another beer or two and take my exit to her apartment. When she brushed her hair back over her ear and rubbed her neck, it meant, "Get your ass to the apartment now; the key is under the mat." When I put my hand on my face, that meant, "Let's get out of here. I'll leave first." I really don't think anyone ever picked up on that elaborate sign language. We never winked, touched, sat together, or did anything else that would give any indication we were seeing each other.

I really liked her a lot, and I was able to talk to her. She knew, full well, the consequences of blabbing about our little situation of "friends with benefits" to anyone in the hospital. And it stayed quiet for three years, but, predictably, she finally did have to tell someone—the worst person she could have ever told—and soon I was part of the rumor mill, big-time. By the time it got back to me, I was physically intimate with an ICU nurse, an ER nurse, a 4 Northwest pulmonary nurse, a social worker, and a physical therapist ... which was all false, except for the ICU nurse. I only *kissed* the rest of them at various times.

So, some very important lessons were learned. When you think it can't happen to you, it can. No matter how much they do not want to tell someone about it, they will. When you think people don't have a clue about what is going on, they do. And, I guess, if none of that bothers you, that's OK ... but in the hospital, it's probably not cool.

Chris left the hospital and moved away to go back to school, but she sure helped me through a lot of tough years during residency. And I don't blame her for leaking any information about us, but, really, who am I kidding? Hell, I'm sure everyone knew anyway. But three years probably remains a record at the hospital till this day.

I sometimes can't help myself when I see a woman brush her hair back over her ear and rub her neck. It does take me back.

Post Hoc

Looking back, I often think about all of the relationships that were formed during those years. Funny thing about stressful environments: Things like that happen. I suspect the reasons they do are many. For me, I enjoyed hanging out with people who understood what I was going through, whom I could talk to, and it was a bonus that the majority of these people were female and easy on the eyes. And I think, by and large, the nurses liked hanging out with us for all of the same reasons.

I try never to pry or be concerned with anyone else's private life…God knows I have had enough of my own shit to deal with, without having to borrow from someone else. I also try never to judge someone; everyone has reasons for what they decide to do, whether or not I agree with them.

Edward Walker, M.D., ultimately got caught by a very angry wife. Now, how many times has that happened in my years of medicine? He was apparently given an ultimatum: move back to his home country with her or become a beggar, because she would have taken everything he had. He opted for the former. In fact, it still pisses me off to this day; he offered me that black Porsche 911 at a great price. I could kick myself today for not buying it. Oh well, there'll be another shit-for-brains M.D. liquidation sale somewhere. I can guarantee it.

Sloane (not her real name) was a very hot young woman. Something about fake tits kind of turns my stomach, but I know that does it for a lot guys. She was one of those young new divorcées who, flush with newfound freedom, screwed absolutely everybody. I don't know how one could have felt very special in her bed, but a lot of the guys I trained with would not give a shit about that. Sloane broke a number of them in. She left the hospital where I trained a couple of years after the incident with Walker. I heard that she ultimately got married, settled down, had a couple of kids, and became a floor nurse. I'll bet she still turns the heads of young interns.

I really tried to avoid the trap of seeing nurses with whom I worked. I just have never thought that was a good situation, yet, I did—and I would like to say that I am sorry I did it, but I really, honestly, cannot. Chris (not her real name) provided support that helped me make it through some very difficult times. She was really one of the sweetest people I have ever known. She demanded nothing. I know that she had been through a bad relationship, and I think I provided some affirmation and promoted a return in her self-confidence, which was destroyed after that bad relationship ended. I guess I was that all-too-important "transitional man" for her. And that's OK with me; I think it was a mutually beneficial time we spent together.

I found myself over the years wanting to try to find her, to talk to her when things were particularly bad for me at various times in my life and career. But I really do not know what happened to her and never found out. I heard she went back to school, for what I am uncertain, but I know she subsequently got married. Someone told me she had a couple of kids, but after the kids came, she had some issues being a mother, wife, and career woman. I hope all of that got straightened out, if it's true. I really hope she is happy. She most certainly deserves it.

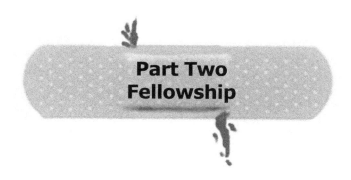

Part Two
Fellowship

Sometimes people are confused about the difference between a resident and a fellow. A fellow has finished his or her residency and is now doing subspecialty training. For example, in internal medicine, sub-specialties exist in lung disease, heart disease, kidney disease, infectious disease, gastrointestinal disease, liver disease, endocrine disease, rheumatologic disease, blood disease, and cancer. A doctor completes an internal-medicine residency and then may opt to practice general internal medicine or to go further and complete a two- to three-year fellowship in a sub-specialty. I chose nephrology (kidney disease).

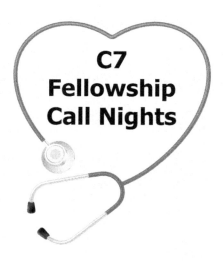

C7
Fellowship Call Nights

I thought that once my internship and residency were over, as I moved into a sub-specialty fellowship, call nights would become much easier. That turned out to be very wrong. The process of learning how to take call starts all over again. My fellowship was completed in a large county-based hospital system, a VA medical center, and a large private hospital. Each was very different, and each had its own little nuances of taking call.

The county hospital system did most all of the indigent care in the area. I can't even tell you how many beds it had; it seemed like a million to me. As a fellow, I was on call every fourth night for my sub-specialty. I thought that these call nights would be easier, being able to take calls from home, but not so. On the majority of my call nights, I remained in the hospital, trying to catch a nap here and there in the fellow sleep room.

There were fellows in every medical sub-specialty, all training at the same time. All of us would have roughly the same call frequency. There were a few call rooms assigned to the fellows, and each of us was given a key. A bathroom across the hallway contained a shower that we all shared, men and women. We also shared the call rooms, which usually had four beds—bunk beds, just like a prison cell. It was first come, first served.

I think that most of the women fellows I met were so focused on medicine, they had little desire for anything else. I know that steely focus made many of them absolute bitches, and they were good at it. And I think that explains, in part, why the majority of them became just like "one of the guys." We all slept in the same call rooms, shared usage of the bathroom, and saw each other on rounds. Frequently, we argued the salient aspects of cases—sometimes to the point of heated discussions culminating in the classic question, "Do you have any literature to back up what you say?" I always interpreted that as meaning, "You are a lying, stupid sack of shit, and I don't believe a fucking thing you are spouting off, unless you prove it to me."

I remember one very busy night on call. I had finished taking care of a lithium overdose, and it was about 3 a.m. The patient was stable and on dialysis. I let the nurse know I was still in house and to call me if there were any problems. I found the call room almost full. Three of the four beds were full, which left me to grab the last one, and I was lucky enough to get the bottom bunk. I had dozed for about fifteen minutes, not quite asleep, when a female cardiology fellow came into the room looking for a spot. All of the beds were full. I closed my eyes and pretended to be asleep, hoping she would leave.

She tapped me on the shoulder. "Hey, Kyle … you awake?"

"Well, I sure as hell am now."

"Move over, I'm sleeping with you. I have to get off my feet. Besides, I'm cold."

Well, what do you say to that? I moved to the edge of the bunk bed, and she got right in bed with me. Now, I'm a pretty big guy and we had to maneuver ourselves into a position where we could get some sleep. Unfortunately, that was on our left sides, "spoon" style. I tried to position my left and right arms to keep them from becoming numb.

She whispered, "Kyle, dammit, let's just get this over with

right now, so we can rest." She sat up, pulled my left arm underneath her pillow, then grabbed my right hand and pulled it up to her chest underneath her arm, placed my hand on her breast, and put her hand over it.

"Don't get any ideas, and don't expect this again anytime soon. This is the only way we can get any sleep."

I didn't say shit, but I felt like saying, "How do you expect me to sleep now?" But I had just remembered what a bitch she had been to me a few days previously, and all of a sudden I felt like I was in bed with my ex-wife. That pretty much squelched any ideas I might have had.

Going to the bathroom and trying to get a shower was always an adventure. The shower was small and at the end of rectangular-shaped bathroom. The toilet was partitioned away from a urinal, and the urinal was partitioned from the lavatory and mirror. The door had a lock on it, but because we all had to use the same bathroom, it was rarely locked, and if it ever was, when the person who locked it came out, they received a complete ration of shit for not sharing. You just became used to walking in and sharing the bathroom with everyone—gives a whole new meaning to "community bathroom."

Occasionally, but not very often, one would walk in on a woman in the shower, on the toilet, or brushing her teeth.

Some were more modest than others and those women preferred the bathrooms less traveled. I have had to go to the bathroom so bad that, regardless of who was in there, I would simply, go to the urinal, and take care of my business, just so that I could keep going and not stop rounds. And a couple of times, some really funny things occurred in that bathroom.

One time I walked in on one of my female colleagues in the shower. I walked in on her not knowing she was in the shower, as it was in the afternoon, and rarely was anyone in the shower in the afternoon. I took a leak, flushed the urinal, and turned around to find her standing naked outside the shower. I really didn't pay that much attention to her until she said, "Hey, Kyle. Will you please hand me that towel?"

"Yeah. OK, sure." I got the towel and handed it to her with my head kind of pointed down. "Hell, don't be that way," she said. "I don't have anything that I'm sure you haven't seen. Listen, I think I felt something in my breast in the shower—can you give it a feel?" She really did look concerned.

Jumping right into a doctor mode, I agreed to do an impromptu breast exam. As she stood there with an exposed breast, with me holding it, another male fellow walked in. He looked stunned, as if he had just walked in on a romantic interlude or was witness to something he was not supposed to witness.

"Hey asshole," she told him, "don't even go there. This is not what you think, and if I hear any of this getting out, I will personally destroy you and your reputation in this hospital! I hope I made myself perfectly clear, Doctor."

His reply was meek: "Oh, I think you did."

While also occurring during residency, it just seemed like the patients we had to deal with during fellowship were always the worst—horribly noncompliant and absolutely coming in at death's doorstep. These people had never seen a doctor preventively but would come into the ER when they didn't feel well. All of the internal-medicine residents and interns took their turn rotating through the ER and would frequently call fellows for consultations.

One night I finally decided to try and take call from home. Predictably, I was called at 2 a.m. about a dialysis patient who was in the ER because she felt weak. The intern did the appropriate lab tests and found that her potassium level was elevated, a frequent occurrence in dialysis patients, especially right before their scheduled outpatient treatments. I asked the intern when she was scheduled to dialyze, and he said at 6 a.m. I thought about it a second; the patient had no electrocardiographic changes consistent with the high potassium level, so there was at least a question in my mind as to whether or not the result was real. So I told the intern to repeat the test, and if it came back elevated to give her a dose of medicine to bring the potassium down, and repeat the test four hours after the dose. I figured that would give me till at least 6:30 a.m.

The intern called me back and this time the patient's potassium level was even higher. I told him that really would be unusual, but he said that was the result he obtained. I told him I was almost to the hospital and I would come examine the woman.

When I examined her in the ER, everything looked fine, but the lab work was just as the intern had told me. All of the sudden, I spotted a family-size bag of potato chips in her belongings.

"Those potato chips pretty good?" I asked.

"Oh, yeah. I eat them all the time."

I replied, "Have you been eating chips tonight?"

"Oh, yes, sir. I figured it would help me pass the time. And since I like salt so much, I decided to make them healthier, so I've been using this salt substitute."

Salt substitute is potassium chloride.

I brought the intern into the room and asked him for the differential diagnosis of hyperkalemia (very high level of potassium in the blood stream, which can be fatal). After he gave me the standard textbook etiologies, I held up the bag of potato chips and salt substitute and said, "Here's a couple more to add to your list."

You could get abused by other fellows and upper-level residents on call nights. One Sunday night, I was asked by the chief surgery resident to do an emergent consult. One of their cholecystectomy (removal of the gallbladder) patients had slipped into renal failure over a three-day period. I used to hate that shit—letting a patient have a problem for a few days, then dumping it in the lap of someone late at night. But that's something that I now understand happens all the time in practice.

I went in and saw this poor old guy, and diagnosed him as suffering from acute inattention by his surgery house staff. I looked at his lab work, which clearly showed a gradual deterioration of his renal function, but with no apparent reason. I examined the patient and found his bladder to be the size of a basketball. He had a Foley bladder catheter in place to drain his urine, and no one had thought to check to see if it was blocked. I wrote the consultation note in the chart, with the recommendation of "Flush the Foley catheter." I couldn't help but stick a little Post-it note on the consult that the chief resident would see, but would not be a part of the medical record: "Next time, watch the lab, examine the patient, and make sure all your hoses are draining."

I then asked the nurse to call the resident and tell him the consult was on the chart with recommendations for him, which he could follow or not. I left. When he saw me the next day, he looked away and never said a word. Remember what I always tell you, the most fragile thing in the world *is* a doctor's ego.

Fellowship nights on call were in some ways different, but in many ways the same. What I realize now is that fellowship call nights prepare you for the real shit coming down the pike when you enter private practice—well, all except for sleeping and bathing with women you don't know. And while that provided momentary diversion, one thing remains: A hatred for call nights starts very early and persists throughout your career.

Post Hoc

Post-doctoral training in residency and fellowship can get a little crazy at times. Some of the crap that went on still seems so bizarre to me. On the one hand, the interaction with fellow residency colleagues is nothing like the relationships with colleagues in private practice, but on the other hand, it starts to approximate these relationships as training draws to a close.

When professional people work in close proximity to one another, especially every day as in residency and fellowship, I really think there are a lot of boundaries that are broken down. We understand much of what the other has been through and is going through because we are all in it as well, going through similar issues and stressors. You really do become like brothers and sisters...and sometimes you argue and fight like them too.

I look back on these particular stories and I have two opinions. One, I think the interactions I had with those two female fellows—in bed and in the shower—were the most abnormal things ever to have occurred in a work environment. But, two, I know those situations were completely harmless, driven by the stress and lack of sleep, and, once the shock passed, I never thought twice about them. Wait a minute; that's not true—maybe I wondered, at the time, if these were solicitations. But when I look back, I don't know if they were or not. And if they were, maybe I was just too stressed out or too much of a dumb ass to recognize it ... realistically, probably both.

When I used to tell women these stories, their immediate reaction is, "Oh my God. These women were hitting on you. You couldn't see that?"

But when I would tell other guys, especially if they were

physicians they would generally say, "Yeah, whatever." If they were "regular" guys, they would generally say, "Hey—you should've hit on them both."

The bottom line is that I am a firm believer that stress and lack of sleep will do funny things to you. Hmmmm ... I wonder what would have happened?

I thought the little cardiology fellow who got into bed with me was really hot. And to be perfectly honest with you, maybe I should have "followed up" on that. But she was *such a bitch* and, specifically, a bitch to me. Sometimes cardiologists and nephrologists don't see eye to eye, and looking back, I can only imagine what a relationship like that would have been like. Oh, wait a minute—yeah...I think I already know.

The other fellow, the one whose breast I fondled—I mean examined—was the nicest woman you could ever want to know. She was, and I'm sure still is, one of the most compassionate women I have ever met, personally or professionally. She is an oncologist and a damn good one. Maybe being an oncology fellow made her pay a little more attention to her own breasts—not to mention the fact that I suspect she had taken care of a breast-cancer patient that day.

Dealing with interns, residents, and other fellows is an art every bit as much as medicine itself is. I trained in a high-powered academic institution, where intimidation was the main mode of teaching. Pretty soon, in a setting like that, everyone is at each other's throat. And now, as I look back, I wish that I had been kinder to those interns, residents, and fellows with whom I worked.

I am a graduate of a medical school that conferred the D.O. degree, instead of the traditional M.D. degree. D.O.'s receive extra training in the musculoskeletal system, which make up the muscles and bones of a person. This involves the use of their hands to diagnosis injury and illness and to encourage the body's natural ability to heal. Osteopathic physicians are more likely to use a patient's first name and to discuss social, family and emotional impact of illness. Other than that there are few differences between D.O.s and M.D.s. Those who do not know this, often think D.O.'s are inferior to M.D.'s because they are not as well trained. I trained with ALL M.D.'s. I had been exposed to some degree of discrimination during my residency, but doing fellowship training amongst ALL M.D.'s in a very large well known academic institution back during those years, was especially intimidating. To be totally honest with you, being designated as a doctor of osteopathic medicine (D.O.) and training with doctors of medicine (M.D.) really put a chip on my shoulder, and I berated the shit out of any of those little fuckers who crossed me. Even though I went to medical school for four years like everyone else and trained in one of the country's most respected academic institutions, many consider me to be an "inferior" physician because my degree is D.O. instead of M.D—and that's a misconception that prevails in the minds of many people even today. Now, I really couldn't give a shit, though I still feel the hair on the back of my neck stand up when I hear things like, "Well, he's not a *real* doctor; he's an old D.O.," but I just consider the source. These people usually obtain their information from a sister or cousin, whichever one they happen to be dating at the time.

If I had it to do over again, I would keep the chip to myself more and be a little kinder. Maybe? Hell, I take that back. In all likelihood, I'd be exactly the same. But I will say this…over the years, that chip on my shoulder gradually went away…today, I actually LIKE having a medical degree that no one else, with whom I work, has. I have worked with some doctors for many years that never even knew my degree was different…and those that did, didn't really care.

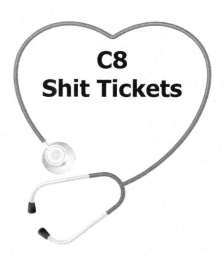

C8
Shit Tickets

Call nights during residency and fellowship had the inherent capability of completely demoralizing, dehumanizing, and degrading a young resident or fellow. Your life is measured in intervals between calls and biologic urges. You eat stale hospital food, listen to the laments of the sick and injured, cater to the day and night calls of nurses in distress or just pissed off, go for a couple of days without bathing or shaving, and when you *can* sleep, it is on a bed that is akin to a prison bunk in a community setting. I look back and it just seems like it was a six-year fraternity hazing incident.

The food was uniformly miserable. The hospital system in which I completed my residency maintained a main cafeteria in the basement and a grill located on the main floor, near the entrance. After the first couple of meals in the cafeteria, it became clear that the grill was the only viable option, but it was like eating bar food without the ability to chase what you were choking down with a cold beer. And the food was totally dependent upon which derelict they had in there doing the cooking. I often wondered, "Where the hell do they find these people and what *are* their qualifications?" One could dine on a hamburger, grilled cheese, or a hot dog, all with the obligatory order of fries—the trans-fatty-acid-laden grease was tossed in at no extra charge.

These gourmet fast-food delights were paid for with meal tickets; we were each given one ticket per call night. And God help you if your meal went one penny over the allotted three-dollar amount, because then you had to deal with Cerberus, the three-headed watchdog from hell, who took great pride in roughing you up. Now that I think about it, she must have taught the nurses. If you didn't have the cash, you either had to burn the meal ticket you had saved from the last night on call, or put back the drink ... there were no other options.

I remember when I decided to not eat in there anymore. We had an outpatient clinic, and hospital employees could be seen there for a reduced price. I was working there one afternoon when one of the derelict grill-dudes who flipped burgers came in. And I was, fortunately or unfortunately, assigned to see him.

"Hey, man, I know you—you're that doctor that eats in the grill," he said when he saw me.

"That's right, sir. What kind of trouble are you having today?"

"Man, my nature be hurting."

"Excuse me?"

"You know, man … my NATURE … my DICK, man," he answered in a very frustrated tone.

I asked him the other pertinent historical questions that go along with attempting to evaluate such a complaint. "OK … let's have a look," I said then.

Well, all I can say is, what do you give the guy who has everything?

The correct answer is: the entire medicine cabinet. He was eaten up with genital herpes, gonorrhea, and either scabies or the viral infection molluscum contagiosum. I didn't stay in the room long enough to determine which of the latter he actually had; the first two were enough. I treated him for everything I could imagine after the cultures were obtained, and then I think I went into the bathroom and puked. This son of a bitch had been fucking feeding us! I just prayed to God that he took to heart that sign in the bathroom that said, "Employees MUST wash their hands before returning to work." Something tells me that wasn't high on his priority list. I never ate in that place again, and I told my good friends about it so they wouldn't eat in there either. But the assholes—them I just let continue, figuring they deserved what they got.

The hospital I worked in during my fellowship, the county system, put a damn McDonald's in the lobby; talk about your conflict of interest. I was told it was one of the busiest in the city. You would see all matter of patients in that place—some pushing IV poles, others carrying Foley catheters with tubes coming out from underneath their gowns, teeming with urine, and still others with outpatient or ER armbands, who decided to grab a quick Mickey D's and then head back for their lab results.

But the idea of trying to eat at all on call nights quickly became unappealing; just one more step in the demoralization process.

Part of becoming a good doctor is to learn how to listen to the moaning, groaning, and complaints of the patient. But sometimes the conversation would simply drag you down, especially after having been up all night. Try discussing bowel habits of alternating constipation and diarrhea with a half-demented eighty-year-old great-grandmother ... or unrelenting flatulence with a little old man who continues to fart during the interview and exam.

One of my favorite consultations was a discussion I had with a sweet little old lady, in which she explained a very interesting little problem with me. "Doctor, I have been having a problem with wet gas."

"I'm sorry Mrs. Greenberg, you said what?"

She repeated it: "I am having a problem with wet gas."

"Mrs. Greenberg, could you explain that a little more in detail to me so that I can understand?"

"Oh, sure. Whenever I pass gas, something else comes out."

"OK ... I think I've got the picture now. I am going to put you on Metamucil and I want you to increase the fiber in your diet; let's see if that doesn't help."

She smiled as if satisfied with the therapy I had prescribed. I didn't have the heart to tell her that the "wet gas" problem she described was, in reality, that she was simply shitting on herself.

One night during my fellowship, I had had all I could take. I had just been bitched out by a hormonal dialysis nurse. I was thirty-six hours into no sleep. I didn't dare eat any food and I was about to shit my pants. I was a broken young doctor, finally hitting rock bottom, wanting nothing more than to simply take a crap in peace. Every time I would get to the point of pulling my pants down, that fucking pager would go off; finally I just had to ignore it. And so there I was, sitting on the john in the community toilet, when one of the other fellows walked in.

He recognized my running shoes underneath the stall. "Hey, Kyle. How's it going?"

"How's it going? You really want to know? I have been up for thirty-six hours straight. I stink. I have just had my ass chewed out by a bitch on the tenth floor. I spent my day trying to be kind to an old man who farted during the entire exam. I followed that up with fighting the uncontrollable desire to frankly tell a little old lady she wasn't having wet gas, she was actually shitting on herself. I can't eat any food because I have visions of a herpetic and gonorrhea-infested penis in the middle of a hot-dog bun. AND I have been trying to take a shit for the past two hours! Taking a shit is the only thing that is remotely satisfying to me at this stage in my life and these mother fuckers have even taken that pleasure away by placing toilet paper in here that you could sand the fucking walls with and that has the absorbent capacity equal to the tile on this fucking floor! Hell, it's more like trying to wipe your ass on a roll of tickets—as a matter of fact, that's what these are ... SHIT TICKETS!"

The other fellow never said a word, but I could see that his feet never moved. I heard the door open again and another fellow walked in and asked, "What the hell is going on in here?"

The first guy calmly replied: "Smith is on the shitter going postal. I think he's lost it this time—and with his pants down on the toilet, how Freudian can you get? Best just to leave him alone."

Then they walked out. Word got out among the residents and fellows, and from that point on the toilet tissue was no longer referred to as such, but as "shit tickets."

They say that individuals must be broken so that they can be rebuilt, and having to wipe my ass with those "shit tickets" marked rock bottom for me. To this day, I do not care how much it costs for the good stuff, my ass will never again be touched by industrial toilet tissue; the memories are too intense—no, sir, only the best and softest will do. I think from that point forward, I was a better doctor, because I couldn't be more demoralized or dehumanized than that. When you are truly at the worst spot, it can only get better. And it did; it's just the call nights never did. Only the ability to handle them improved steadily.

Post Hoc

You know, I still laugh out loud when I read this chapter. I swear to you, it was like it happened yesterday. I really believe that before an intern, resident, or fellow can really become a good doctor, he or she must hit rock bottom … and by that, I mean that he or she must come to the realization that not all of medicine is glamour and glory. It is damn hard work that takes a lot out of you. It is humbling and it teaches you very quickly that as smart as you think you are, you do not know everything and you cannot save everyone.

The wise physician knows that part of his job is to hold someone's hand, and to not get upset or put out because a patient doesn't understand something you've said. What may seem the most mundane, trivial complaint to you might actually be an indication of a patient's fear that is near panic level; you see "mundane," but they're in fear of their health or life. I think that a lot of physicians never learn that lesson. I know them; I hear what they say about patients who "bother" them. I don't look at it that way. I am here to help, to ease pain and suffering, and if that means holding the hand of a little old lady who shit her pants, then that's what it means. But I don't think a lot of doctors learn that.

I have learned those lessons at this point in my career. The little old man with flatulence, the little old lady with "wet gas," the lack of sleep, the confrontation with the dialysis nurse—they all happened at one point. If you believe things happen for a reason—and I'm not sure if I do or do not—then you would have to say that all of those things happened to help me realize my mission on this earth as a doctor. Getting to that point in my training was necessary for me to progress. And it made me a better doctor.

Too bad this cannot be taught in medical school.

Part Three
Private Practice

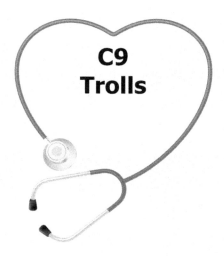

C9
Trolls

There are some people you would just rather not have to deal with. That certainly rings true in the practice of medicine. While one could be led to believe that physicians love dealing with *all* people, being the humanitarians we uniformly are (now that even makes ME laugh), we are also human, and being human lends itself to having to do crap you really do not want to do, for people you really do not want to do it for.

However, this perspective changed for me within the first few years of call nights. Inevitably, people will ignore things all day long, waiting for the most inopportune time to call a physician or go to the local emergency room for help—usually between the hours of 10 p.m. and 3 a.m. Now, I'm the first to admit that certain problems can present at any time of the day or night, and in unexpected fashion, and taking care of people who need to be taken care of emergently has never been an issue for me—that is why I am here, and it is my pleasure to help them. I am specifically referring to those patients who assume no responsibility for their own care, have no regard for the health-care professionals who must assume that responsibility for them, and who are, frankly, just downright disgusting people to have to deal with anyway.

I learned during call nights that you can develop ... well, just a nasty feeling for some of the more disgusting of these people. I also learned the term to describe them quickly—*trolls*—and I am referring to the scary things that live under bridges, not the fishing technique.

In many hospitals, the trolls are widely known. They inhabit the same area and, predictably, will show up at the same time. One learns very early in one's medical career that as soon as you start to think, "I haven't seen so-and-so in a while," or, "I wonder whatever happened to so-and-so," invariably the trolls sense this and make immediate, spectacular returns. The names of the trolls who survive over a period of time are even handed down among house staff, generation to generation. And the fun doesn't stop with internship, residency, and fellowship; it even gets better in private practice.

The list of trolls goes on to, seemingly, infinity. The troll gene never breeds itself out of the population, and there will always be a never-ending supply of them. Here are a few of my personal favorites from my fellowship training.

Mary was fifty-five years old, morbidly obese—frankly a fat-ass—woman, chronologically. Her body was closer to that of a ninety-five-year-old. Having abused herself for years and years, she was now left to deal with the ravages of congestive heart failure, diabetes, and chronic lung disease. I guess she just figured out that her time on this earth was not very long, so she continued to do what she liked to do—and that was smoke at least four packs of cigarettes a day and eat like a pig. She had seen multiple hospitalizations for her lung ailment, presenting with shortness of breath, pneumonia or bronchitis, and a touch of heart failure tossed in for good measure. She would come into the hospital; go off the cigarettes for a few days; get IV antibiotics, respiratory therapy, and a few hot meals; and go home: It was like a spa treatment for the old bat. Every time this happened, we had a detailed conversation about the cigarettes and how they were killing her, and each time she would just say, "Hell, Doc, I know. And I promise you, I'm gonna quit."

One of these hospital stays lasted a little longer than I had expected, and I just could not figure out why. She seemed to do better, responding to the treatment, but then she'd start wheezing again despite the therapy that was prescribed for her. I was lamenting this to a nurse while writing my notes one day.

The nurse remarked, "You know she's smoking again."

"What?" She usually quit while she was admitted, (getting toned up). "Are you sure?"

"Yeah," the nurse said. "I caught her myself. I thought she was going to blow us all to kingdom come, smoking in the room next to the oxygen. She was standing at the window, holding the oxygen tubing in the same hand she was holding the lit cigarette. She would take a drag and blow the smoke out the window."

"No shit," I said. "Thanks. I'll take care of this."

I stormed into Mary's room to find her watching her soap operas and eating a candy bar. "Mary, we need to talk."

"Not now, Doc. You know I can't be disturbed when I'm watching my shows."

I reached up and turned the television off.

"Now dammit, Doc. You've gone too far this time."

I interrupted her: "Mary, we've known each other for a while now. You know you're killing yourself with the cigarettes. You know not to smoke in the hospital. I've been busting my ass to get you better and you smoke in the room with oxygen going? You can kill yourself if you want to, but don't take any of us with you."

She was really angry now. "You accusing me of something, you son of a bitch?

"Yeah, I am. Want me to go get the nurse who caught you? She's lying, or you are—hell, I'll just go get her right now!" I started out the door.

"Hey … wait a minute," Mary called me back. "OK, OK. I'm sorry I called you a son of a bitch. OK, I did it."

I just said, "OK. Don't try to bullshit me again. And give me the cigarettes … NOW!"

"Awwww Doc, let me keep 'em. It's my last pack."

Shaking my head, I just said, "Uh-uh … NOW, Mary."

She rolled out of bed, lifted her gown to expose the largest breasts I had ever seen, raised her left one up off her thigh, and pulled the pack of cigarettes and lighter out from underneath it with the other hand. I watched this performance, flabbergasted.

"Here you go." She tried to hand me the pack of cigarettes and lighter.

I told her to leave them on the nightstand, and the nurse would come get them. That's a hell of a cigarette case, isn't it?

I have had to take care of patients with all manner of

psychiatric disorders in my years, some with very bizarre thought processes and habits. One guy, a forty-two-year-old man, would come into the hospital about every two to three weeks with intractable nausea, vomiting, and diarrhea. He received the million-dollar work-up not once, but twice. After a few days of IV fluids and bowel rest, he would return to normal. I must have talked to that guy a hundred times, desperately trying to find the exact cause.

One day on rounds, I decided I would call his psychiatrist and try to get a little more insight. The psychiatrist told me the patient had a strange obsessive-compulsive disorder, and he fixated on starvation; he was intensely afraid of going without food. I then called the half way house this guy lived in and asked if I could come look around. They were very accommodating to me, showing me the dining facilities and the patient's room.

When I walked into his room, I noticed a very pungent odor, frankly disgusting, like food that had gone bad in a refrigerator, but there *was* no refrigerator. I followed the stench to a chest of drawers. I opened the top drawer to find a dozen half-eaten bologna sandwiches in bags, molded bread, all of it in stages of decomposition. He was stealing food from the dining room, taking it to his room, hiding it, and eating on it for days—effectively giving himself a nice case of food poisoning every couple of weeks.

Another patient, Debra, was a frequent flyer—a thirty-four-year-old, brittle diabetic who refused to take care of herself. She had all the ravages of diabetes, and she smoked, which made everything worse. She had lost half of one foot from diabetes; she couldn't feel anything and developed what I thought was a vascular insufficiency ulcer on the sole of her foot. It got infected, then the bone got infected, and she ultimately needed a trans-metatarsal amputation.

She was back in the hospital the following year with another of these things on the same stump, but it was in a strange position. On the way out of the hospital one evening, I saw her outside in her hospital gown, barefoot, walking on the stump without a bandage, and smoking the last part of her cigarette. She didn't see me; I just stood and watched. When she finished her cigarette, she tossed it on the ground, and stamped out the flame with her bare stump. Since she couldn't feel anything, she couldn't feel the flame of the cigarette underneath her foot, or what was left of it. I recommended a below-the-knee amputation at that point—why carve her up? Just take it off so she could at least walk, and she could stamp her cigarette out with her prosthesis.

I especially loved it when a whole family of trolls would get into the act and rally around the sickest of the bunch.

Sometimes they would get into little arguments. Janie was a very sweet lady, but fat as a hog and married to the skinniest man I ever saw. She was twenty-eight years old, had a couple of kids, and a rip-roaring case of high blood pressure and diabetes. She had tattoos all over her arms—multiple names of men and a few scars where she had gotten so pissed at some of them that she had the tattoo just cut off. The worst one was between her legs on the inner aspect of her thigh, a homemade tattoo that said, "Raymond's Pussy" with an arrow drawn toward her vagina. I think Raymond was her ex-husband, but I was never really very sure about that. And I suppose it didn't matter anyway, because Raymond forever claimed that territory as his own.

Janie would go off her medications and come in with diabetic keto-acidosis and emergent hypertension, and she did so frequently. Many times she would just run out of her medicines and wouldn't bother to go get refills. She blamed her skinny little husband, Johnny, and Johnny blamed her. Go figure. During one of these hospitalizations, Janie's parents came to visit and I had the misfortune of making rounds during the time they were there. Between Janie, Johnny and her parents there was not a full set of teeth in the room. When I explained the chronic problems she had and that she would continue to have serious problems if she did not take her medications, the father wanted to talk with me—in private. I agreed reluctantly—because I had learned that whenever that happens, it is *not* going to be a good conversation.

We stepped outside the room. "Doc," he began. "I ain't gonna lie to ya. My baby is being kilt by that skinny little sumbitch in there. I wanted to whip him to fried whale shit, but the old lady'll kick my ass and me out the goddamn house if I do. But I'm telling ya that he ain't gettin' her medicines. He don't do shit for her. Let me tell ya what the little motherfucker did last Thanksgivin'. We's all goin' over to Janie's for Thanksgivin' and give thanks to the Lord for all he's done for us. She had the table already sat. We went over there and just went right on in the house like we always do. Doc, he had my baby up on that table banging the shit outta her, right there on the Thanksgivin' table where we's gonna give thanks to the Lord. I'm a tellin' ya, Doc, he's a sick sumbitch …"

I was not a bit surprised.

Like I said, trolls will always be in never-ending supply … and a necessary hazard to negotiating call nights.

Post Hoc

Now the term "trolls" is very derogatory, I admit … but it is *so* appropriate. Please do not misunderstand me. I sincerely believe that there is not one person on this earth who is any better than anyone else, so I am, in no way, attempting to say that I am better than trolls. Let's just say that I think I respect others who must care for me more than trolls do, and maybe I assume a little more responsibility for my health; perhaps my bartender would think otherwise, but I tip the hell out of him, so I'm sure he would swear that I *do* take good care of myself. At least, if he knows what's good for him.

Mary (not her real name) tormented me throughout my fellowship. I really liked her; I just didn't like how she treated herself. I have seen a lot of breasts in my professional career, and I have seen a lot of really shocking and frankly gross things, but I must say that the episode with Mary retrieving the contraband cigarettes and lighter from underneath her pendulous breasts was an all-time low. She died a few years after this story happened; there's only so much a body can take.

The schizophrenic man with the food issue was a very interesting case. I learned how to pay attention to detail from this case, and it still remains one of my best diagnostic accomplishments. I just figured there was more to this case than met the eye. And I learned, also, that sometimes a doctor needs to play detective and look under a few rocks; you'd be surprised what you'll find.

I really don't know what to tell you about Janie (not her real name), truly one of the most bizarre people I have ever seen. Her family and situations were just as strange. These people truly lived from one biologic urge to the next. Not many family discussions have left me speechless, but this one truly did. Janie died shortly after this admission; she stopped taking her medicine again. Hell, maybe Johnny (not his real name, either) had something to do with it. She came in with massive cerebral stroke—it was hopeless, and she could not be saved. I have always remained sad about that.

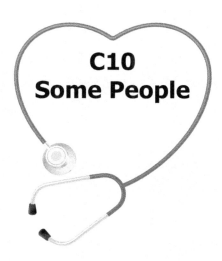

C10
Some People

One of the most difficult things to learn and deal with on call nights is being required to take care of those patients who refuse to take care of themselves. These are patients who, for whatever reason, refuse to take their medicine, do not follow their doctor's advice, or miss life-saving treatments. They invariably show up in the middle of the night in some sort of extremis, requiring the unlucky soul on call that night to jump in and save their asses and then generally to return another day as a repeat offender.

I have often wondered what causes someone to go to the doctor, get advice, and obtain medicine to improve the quality of his life, only to refuse to take either the medicine or any responsibility for his own health and well-being. After observing these types of patients over the years, I have come to the following conclusion: Patients who are stricken with any type of chronic disease or illness, especially when that disease or illness occurs in childhood or young adulthood, lose a certain amount of control over their lives. Their lives become dictated by what they can and cannot do, what they can and cannot eat, what they can and cannot drink—all of this to the point that they have lost any semblance of "self." In certain of these patients, refusing to take medications or show up for treatments— basically to being noncompliant— is, simply, their way of exercising the only control they have over their lives.

And there is another subset of these patients, those who are cared for by family members or others who are close to them. These patients become the central focus of the family because of their illness. In many circumstances, these patients make a subconscious connection between their disease and receiving the love and attention they so desperately need. The illness, then, becomes vital to their survival, and the thought pattern becomes "take the illness away, love and attention goes away, and I will be left alone." When this kind of thinking, conscious or subconscious, is present, there is little a doctor can do to make the patient better.

Still, even though we can understand some of the thought patterns, processes, and pathology of these poor patients, that does not mitigate how absolutely pissed off the on-call doctor can get with being repeatedly called out to pull their asses out of the fire. We all have to do it, and we all have "favorites." The trick is getting pissed off and then letting it go. You cannot change them. You cannot help them. And sometimes things are not always the way you think they are. Here are a few of my favorites.

Joseph was a thirty-one-year-old guy who had suffered from diabetes for most of his life. Stricken with the disease in early childhood, he progressed to develop near-blindness; neuropathy, a complication where he lost sensation in his feet except an intense burning pain; and kidney failure requiring dialysis. He was a very angry person, angry at everyone and everything. Joseph frequently refused to take his insulin or to follow his fluid restriction, and he missed his dialysis treatments. So he'd present to the hospital nearly dead, a metabolic mess, with fluid in his lungs requiring him to be placed on a ventilator and admitted to the ICU, and needing emergent dialysis to save his life. This drill occurred with some regularity—three times a month, to be exact.

Joe had a girlfriend who was also in bad shape—crippled from childhood, requiring large metal braces and crutches to help her walk. She loved him with all her heart, even though he treated her like shit. She had a bad habit of falling, and when she did, it sounded like two metal trash cans being tossed down a concrete alleyway. There were a couple of times I heard that sound and immediately knew Joe was in the house.

I happened to be the unlucky guy on call for each of Joseph's admissions one month; on three different call nights, I took care of him all night long. On his third admission, I transferred him to the floor after he was dialyzed and extubated (taken off the mechanical ventilator). On evening rounds the next day, I stopped by to have a little chat with Joe and his girlfriend, Janie. Joe was not a very pleasant person to be around, and I was still pissed off for having to take care of him all month.

"Dammit, Joe—you realize you are on the fast track to killing yourself? Not to mention what you're doing to Janie AND to me."

He looked away, wouldn't make eye contact with me, and said nothing. I continued berating him.

"If you want to kill yourself, you go right ahead and do it. Just don't do it on my watch. Hell, I'm tired of this shit. Why don't you just put a fucking gun to your head; it's a lot quicker."

At this point Janie started crying. "Joe, listen to Doc. He's just trying to take care of you. Please!"

Joe just shrugged his shoulders and sat, without a sound.

"OK, Joe, here's the plan. I'm going to send the nurses in here to put you in the shower and give you a bath. You stink."

It was only this that actually got a response out of him. He quickly looked up at me, very angry. "I ain't takin no shower, man."

"Oh yes, you are. And if you give the nurses any shit whatsoever when they get in here to bathe you, I will come back and bodily pick your scrawny ass up and bathe you myself. And I won't be quite as gentle as they will be. Don't you fuck with me, Joe … I mean it."

Janie cried harder and harder. Joe asked, "Why are you treating me like this, man?"

"Because you can't take care of yourself, Joe."

I turned around and walked out of the room to Janie's sobs, only to hear her falling out of her chair—the sound of the damn trash cans being tossed down the alley.

Joseph came in one more time after that admission. This time he wasn't so lucky. He died in the ER, despite everything everyone did to save him. We just couldn't save Joe from himself, and maybe he wanted it that way. I was told Janie was beside herself with grief. And I have to admit, I was sad too when I found out that Joe had died, maybe reflecting on my own failure to get anything across to him. I felt badly for having berated him as I did. Maybe Joe forgave me for that ... but I suspect he didn't.

Another of my little darlings was Lisa. She was in her mid-thirties and had man-eating high blood pressure, the worst I ever saw. We spent well over a million dollars on her, trying to get to the bottom of her blood-pressure problem. You name it, we studied it, X-rayed it, and looked for every known cause of it. We found nothing, and were relegated to treating it with high doses of four different drugs.

The problem with a couple of these drugs was that the patient could get rebound high blood pressure if they were abruptly stopped, and guess what Lisa would do? Frequently. It was a predictable occurrence toward the end of the month, when the prescriptions she was sent home with from the last hospitalization started running out. And it ALWAYS happened at night. She would come in with a condition called hypertensive crisis; she would present with disorientation and combativeness, deteriorate to a seizure, and have a blood pressure somewhere between 260 and 280 millimeters of mercury, systolic, and somewhere between 120 and 160 millimeters of mercury, diastolic—very high in anyone's book. We would be up all night bringing it down slowly, until she was calm and the blood pressure was in a livable range. She would get transferred to the floor the next day, started on her oral medicines, and then she'd leave the hospital when no one was looking, signing out AMA (against medical advice). This happened every time. I got to the point that I just left her prescriptions in her room, hoping she would take them with her—sometimes she did, but most times she didn't.

Lisa was very sweet when I talked with her. She would always tell me she was sorry she ran out of her medicines, and she'd vow *never to do it again*. I think she meant well, but there was a disconnect there somewhere. Finally she came in one night with a huge intra-cerebral hemorrhage—the kind you don't survive. Her skull was full of blood; all we could do was place her on the ventilator, waiting until we could officially declare brain death. I liked Lisa; she just didn't like herself, and I have to admit I was heartbroken when I discontinued life support and pronounced her dead.

Other times, patients would come in late at night in trouble, and we would assume that their own noncompliance was the culprit. I always remembered what "they" say about what happens when you "assume"? That's right, you make an "ass" out of "u" and "me." Well, one night I made the biggest ass out of myself *ever*—and for me to say that, *about me*, reveals an awful lot. That night, I felt the worst I have ever felt in my life.

I was called to the ER to see a little old lady who missed her dialysis treatment. She was in pulmonary edema (fluid in the lungs), her potassium was very high, and she needed to be emergently dialyzed at 2 a.m. I was *so pissed*. I was determined to teach her a lesson—the audacity she had, to skip a treatment and inconvenience me and the dialysis nurse. When I walked into the room, I found this little old lady, eighty-two years old, who could have been my grandmother. My anger level immediately went down a notch. She was very soft-spoken and, although she was in respiratory distress and clearly uncomfortable, she did not complain, only simply answered my questions.

"Mrs. Greer, don't you know that you have to go to dialysis? If you do not go to dialysis, the fluid will build up in your lungs and you cannot breathe, and it will ultimately kill you. When you decide not to go to dialysis, it's a decision that affects a lot of people. You inconvenience me, but worse than that, I have to call a dialysis nurse out specifically to take care of you. Now why wouldn't you have gone to dialysis today?"

After this lecture from me, she had big tears rolling out

of her eyes. In a low, contrite voice, she spoke words that pierced me to my soul. "Doctor, I am so sorry. I would never do anything to put anyone out. I know you are busy and you could be doing other things than taking care of this old lady, and I will apologize to the dialysis nurse. My husband of sixty-four years has terminal pancreatic cancer. He isn't doing very well. I knew he would die today. And I have just been with him for so long, I couldn't leave him."

I wiped the tears from my eyes, patted her hand, and left the room to write her orders. I NEVER ask anyone why they don't do what they are supposed to do anymore.

Post Hoc

Now I know, at this point, you must be thinking that I think all patients are idiots and, were it not for me, they would all die horrible deaths in quite short order.

That is only partially true.

As I try to teach patients how to be more responsible about taking care of themselves, I have found over the years that the patients actually teach me much more than I could ever teach them. Some of the lessons I learn are about medicine, some of them are about life, and some of them are about me.

I learned a most significant lesson when I confronted that old lady. Not everything is as it appears. I can honestly say that this still hurts my heart—that I could think only about me, and not about the welfare and good of the patient. I have often wondered what happened to her and whether she ever forgave me for that encounter when I was less than kind to her. I hope she would have forgiven me, but if it were me in her position, I am not sure I'd be that generous. I hope she is in a better place, with no more suffering.

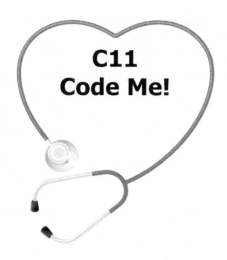

C11
Code Me!

I have had the distinct pleasure—or displeasure, as it were—of observing all manner of familial interactions on call nights. These interactions range from the most loving, understanding, and intense to the most dysfunctional, ignorant, and bizarre, sometimes all within the same family. I find it absolutely fascinating to watch. There is nothing easier than explaining a situation to an intelligent family member, who asks all the right questions, and accepts the reasonable outcomes associated with their loved one's illness. On the other hand, there is nothing more difficult than trying to explain something to someone who will not listen and has an inherent distrust of you and, for that matter, all doctors.

I believe there is a way to talk with all people, regardless of educational level socioeconomic status, or intelligence. There are ways to make people understand whatever you are trying to impart to them. Sometimes it takes a lot of work, but it can be accomplished. I find that one must be flexible and find ways of explaining a concept in a variety of ways; when you work at it, it becomes easier to do. You have to paint a broad picture that can be easily understood. There are those people with whom you can converse on a very high level and they usually want more information. And then others must be spoken with on a very primitive level, and they may not ask any questions at all. The bottom line is that everyone needs to be on the same page in terms of understanding reasonable outcomes.

The worst scenario is being required to talk to multiple family members, which can be a real pain in the ass. I learned to make rounds very early in the morning to avoid relatives altogether, opting to speak with them by phone if necessary. If that doesn't work, I tell them I will meet with them in a conference room so that everyone hears the same message, at the same time. In certain circumstances I have had to tell the family to pick a spokesman, and I agree to communicate with that one person. It really is amazing how several people can be told the *exact same thing* and each come away with a completely different understanding.

I especially loved it when the patient and the family fought over the direction of care. Now, how crazy is that? I mean, it should be up to the *patient*, right? At least that's what I was always taught. You would be surprised how often this occurs. Here is my favorite story about bizarre interactions along this line.

Mr. Lawrence was a sixty-three-year-old man with multiple medical problems. He had diabetes, heart disease, and kidney failure. He was admitted to a small community hospital for what was suspected to be a heart attack. During his hospital stay he developed what seemed to be kidney failure. The small hospital did not offer dialysis services, so he was transferred to the larger hospital where I was training. And he came in on my call night.

He was a big man, but the debilitation of his disease had left him looking much older, and frail. You could tell he had lived a hard life and had probably been a big tough guy when he was younger. He had tattoos all over, most of them homemade. I examined him when he arrived and found him to be in heart failure. His lab work showed that he had, in fact, developed kidney failure at the other hospital. I suspected this was secondary to a combination of underlying diabetes, high blood pressure, and a poorly functioning heart pump that couldn't get enough blood to the kidneys. I started him on some medicine to help his heart pump better, and some high-dose diuretics to jump-start the kidneys in making urine so that we could get the fluid off his lungs.

I went to the waiting room and met his wife. Mrs. Lawrence looked every bit as rough and hard as her husband. She was large, sporting a number of her own tattoos. I explained what had happened and the treatment we were undertaking. I also told her that if the medicine didn't work, we would have to consider dialysis. She seemed to understand everything. The next day Mr. Lawrence had not responded to the medication as I had hoped. I really saw no other option but to try to dialyze him. I was very concerned because with his heart attack a few days before, I knew he had underlying coronary disease. His echocardiogram—an ultrasound test of the heart to measure its ability to pump, among other things—showed that he had an ejection fraction (the percentage of blood ejected out of the heart to the rest of the body) of about 20 to 25 percent, normal being around 60 percent or better.

I explained everything to Mr. Lawrence and his wife, and they agreed to proceed. I placed a central venous dialysis catheter, and we started dialysis. He didn't tolerate it well—actually, not at all—and he coded. Luckily I was right there, and started CPR and got him into ventricular fibrillation, buzzed the hell out of his chest, and got him started right back up again. The dialysis nurse looked at me with a really angry glare.

"WHAT? OK, I know what you're thinking. The answer is no, we are not going to try it again. There, happy?" She smiled and left the room.

I told Mrs. Lawrence what had happened. She was very calm about the whole thing. I explained that we needed to study her husband's heart and hopefully find a blockage we could do something about, but that would commit him to dialysis. She seemed hesitant to move forward, but reluctantly agreed.

I contacted one of the cardiology boys, and he was all too eager to perform a cardiac catheterization on this guy. He went to the cardiac lab almost immediately, and they found a right coronary lesion they were able to angioplasty or open up the blood vessel with a balloon and insert a stent (a small woven metal device that assists the blood vessel in staying open). But the cardiologist told me he wasn't optimistic it was going to help very much because Mr. Lawrence still had a worn-out pump and he had multiple small-vessel disease that could not be angioplastied or bypassed. Basically, he was up a shit creek with no paddle. Still, Mr. Lawrence did OK through the night, and we took him off the ventilator the next morning. I decided to leave well-enough alone and try dialysis again the next day, hoping the cardiologist had fixed the most pressing problem.

The next day, I asked Mrs. Lawrence to come into the room to have a little chat with me and her husband. I explained the whole scenario to them, specifically how dangerous dialysis might continue to be. I broached the subject of life support and CPR should his heart stop again. The conversation that ensued was one of the most interesting patient/family interactions I have ever had.

"I want to let you both know that this could be very risky. Your heart may stop again, and there is no guarantee I can get it started again. I will have to put you back on the ventilator and life support. I need to know before we start what you would want me to do. Some people do not want to be coded and placed on life support, and I just need to know what you want me to do if that happens again."

Nothing was said for a couple of seconds, as they made eye contact with one another. Then Mrs. Lawrence said, "If his heart stops, I think you should just let him go and not put him on the ventilator. Let nature take its course."

Mr. Lawrence quickly interjected: "Now wait just a goddamn minute here. Don't listen to what that bitch says. CODE

ME! I WANT TO BE CODED!"

She quickly replied, "He's just saying that. Don't do anything."

"BULLSHIT!"

I stopped the argument right there. "OK … OK … Let's settle down. OK, Mr. Lawrence, if that's what you want, that's what I'll do. Mrs. Lawrence, I have to do what he wants me to do."

"Well, why the fuck did you pull me in here to begin with?" And with that, she stormed out of the room.

I left to arrange dialysis, and I sat in the ICU and laughed, recounting the patient's old lady saying "let him go" and the patient screaming "CODE ME!" That was just too funny.

Mr. Lawrence made it ok through the dialysis treatment and did well for a few days, but he suffered another heart attack while he was in the hospital. We transferred him back to the ICU and tried to stabilize him. His heart really was just mush, and predictably, he coded again. This time his heart wouldn't restart, and I pronounced him dead. When I notified Mrs. Lawrence that her husband had passed away despite everything I could do, she wailed and wailed uncontrollably, as if she had lost her best friend and lover of many years. And this was the lady who had said "let him go" a few days earlier. I didn't expect her grief response.

I've always scratched my head over that one—I doubt I will ever really figure out her reaction, other than to chalk it up to guilt.

After that call night, I never ask the patient's family what they want done—that is, if the patient can speak for himself. Don't *ever* assume everyone wants the same thing.

Post Hoc

After all these years, the incident with the Lawrence's remains one of the most bizarre and funny interactions I have ever experienced. As I reflect, I think Mr. and Mrs. Lawrence probably had one of those love/hate relationships during the better part of their marriage. There must have been something there because, as I recall, they were married many years.

Now, marriage is a very interesting interaction between two people in and of itself...I've never been good at it, but I would be remiss if I did not comment on it after relating this interaction.

I am reminded of a book written by Jerry M. Lewis, M.D., titled *Marriage as a Search for Healing*. Among other things, the book centers on the question, "Why is it we choose a particular mate?" A very intriguing question, don't you think? After all, the majority of us might say there are any number of people with whom we could have cast our lot ... but what made us choose that one in particular? Dr. Lewis surmises that we choose our mates based on what they do for us psychologically, in that they help us heal from past psychological hurts.

In addition, Dr. Lewis outlines two major issues that must be negotiated to the mutual satisfaction of each partner—if not, there may be animosity that develops as one partner is not fully afforded that to which he or she believes he or she is entitled.

The first of these two issues is the amount of closeness and the amount of separateness which are to be enjoyed in the relationship. In some relationships, the partners spend close to one hundred percent of their time together; others, less; still others, much less. And "closeness" refers not only to the amount of physical intimacy, but also the amount of emotional intimacy that will be enjoyed within the relationship.

The next thing that must be negotiated is the power distribution within the relationship. How will decisions be made—who "wears the pants" in the family? Decision-making can also be one hundred percent one way, zero percent the other, or, again, anything in between.

When I think of these things, I remember the Lawrence

family ... and Dr. Lewis' book. I believe that even dysfunctional couples can stay married if they have negotiated these issues to the mutual satisfaction of the partners. Now I am not so naive as to believe that these are the only things required for a successful relationship, but I do think they're extremely important. But what do I know? As I have admitted many times before, that particular area of human relations has not been my forte.

Funny, because I always thought it would be.

Medicine affords the physician an inner look at the dynamic of human relationships...this, my friend, is an extreme privilege, despite what we sometimes say or think. Learning about the dynamic which governs not only husband and wife interactions, but also familial interactions can be of invaluable assistance to the physician in planning health care option or dealing with end of life issues. For ALL young physicians, those in the health profession, those thinking about entering the field, or people who are privileged enough to be allowed in to witness or observe this interplay, NEVER take it for granted. Take the time to know the patient and the family...it's good medicine.

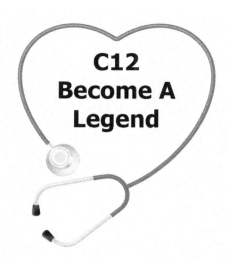

C12
Become A Legend

Just in case you haven't figured it out yet, call nights can be a pain in the ass. They're akin to running a marathon every third or fourth weekend of every month. You have to pace yourself. It's helpful to have little perks during these most miserable times—maybe just a quick stop between hospitals for a soft drink or a new CD to listen to while driving. I discovered another little diversion that was different, but it's not taught in medical schools these days. It's not without hazards, but it can make you feel pretty good, and it gives you the essence of what it really means to be a doctor. I am talking about the forgotten art of house calls.

Many of us are much too young to remember a time

when a doctor would actually come out to the house when someone was sick. He would show up with his stethoscope and medical bag of tricks, maybe leave some pills or pop you in the ass with a slug of penicillin. Sometimes he'd sit in the living room or kitchen and have a glass of iced tea or a cup of coffee, engage in conversation about the family, and then head to the next stop. That was back when people still believed that doctors were placed on this earth to heal and to help others—not merely as objects of malpractice assaults for poor outcomes.

A number of years ago, while on call, I received a message to phone an older lady who was concerned about her husband. He was feeling quite ill, and she said that he could not get out of bed. I explained to her the best option was to call the fire-department paramedics and they would transport him to the local ER, where I would meet them and examine him. She reluctantly agreed. A couple of hours later I phoned the ER and asked if the patient had come in yet; he hadn't. I called the lady back and asked if she had followed my instructions.

"Doctor, I'm sorry, but he is just too stubborn and refuses to come to the hospital," she told me. "I'm worried about him because he says he is too short of breath to get out of the bed, but he says that he is not going to the hospital. I don't know what to do."

It was early evening, and I thought to myself, "This guy is going to come in at 1 a.m. in bad shape, and I'm going to have to drag my ass out of bed to come take care of him. I just know it." At that point, I reasoned that I really wasn't too far from where they lived, and I recalled the days of the forgotten house calls. To be perfectly honest, I thought I could save myself a little late-night work by examining this guy now rather than when he inevitably showed up later. And if he did come into the ER later, at least I would have a good feel for what kind of shape he was in. I thought it would be the humanitarian thing to do. So I asked directions to their house.

The woman, puzzled, asked, "Why do you want to know where we live?"

"I just thought since he would not come see me, I would come see him." She reluctantly gave me directions.

When I showed up, I noticed that their house was in a very bad neighborhood. It was rundown, the yard was unkempt, and the house had burglar bars on the windows and doors. I walked up to the front door and knocked. I heard someone come to the door and knew they were looking at me through the peephole.

"Who is it?" a female voice asked.

"Dr. Smith, Ma'am. I'm the doctor you spoke with on the phone."

She opened the door, looked me over carefully, and asked me in. The house was as unkempt as the yard—old furniture everywhere, pictures of family on every wall, and an old black-and-white television prominently displayed in the living room with rabbit ears for an antenna.

"He's in there," she said, pointing to a front bedroom.

I smiled and nodded. "Thank you, Ma'am."

I found an old man sitting in a bedside rocking chair, looking bewildered as he saw me coming in.

"Who the hell are you? What the hell are you doing in my bedroom?"

I quickly tried to calm him down. "Sir, I'm Dr. Smith. I'm on call this weekend. Your wife called me and said you were very sick and refused to come to the hospital. I offered to come to you instead. How are you feeling?"

"I never felt better," he told me. "The wife's a fucking lunatic and don't know what she's talking about. Now why don't you just tear your ass out of my bedroom and get off my property."

Realizing the situation was deteriorating quickly, I quickly said, "Sir, I'm just a doctor and I meant no harm. I'll be leaving right now."

I walked toward the front door; his wife just stared at me. I felt as if I were in the Twilight Zone. I gave her my card and told her that her husband wanted no part of seeing me and had asked me to leave; she could take him to the hospital if he got ill. She never said a word, but she slammed the door as I walked out, and I could hear her briskly throwing on all of the locks.

Apparently, she took my license-plate number and called the police. She reported me as an intruder and said I entered their home, looked around, frightened them, and left. As I was heading back to the hospital, I was pulled over by two police cars, had a gun leveled at me, was told to put my hands where they could be seen, and then told to walk to the back of the car. They frisked me, cuffed me without telling me what the problem was, and then turned me around as they looked at my ID. They asked me if I had been at the home of these people. I said yes and explained to them that I was a physician on call for my group, and was only making a house call because the woman had told me her husband was short of breath, too ill to get to the hospital, and refused to be transported by the paramedics.

As the officers were checking out my ID and my story, another group of officers came upon the scene. I immediately recognized one of them as a good friend from my ER days. I still treated him and his wife frequently *and* I had recently taken a weekend trip with them to New Orleans. He saw me and his eyes got as big as saucers. "Kyle?" he asked. "What the hell is going on?"

I explained the whole thing to him, and he went back to tell the other officers. They quickly took the cuffs off and vehemently apologized. We all laughed our asses off ... well, I laughed as much as I could after having a gun pointed at me. As they were looking back on the multiple times "suspicious people" calls had come in from that neighborhood, they found that this woman had called and reported break-ins almost every other day. But on investigation, there were never any signs of anything amiss. Talk about your case of mistaken identity.

Thankfully, not all house-call experiences have been that way for me. One time, I decided to make a house call in a slum section of town—a little black lady was feeling very ill and had missed dialysis. Her family was quite concerned and didn't know what to do. I was near them so I decided to make a house call; they were floored when I told them that it would be quicker if I just came to see her. I received directions from them and was at the house in about twenty minutes.

Apparently, even in that short a time, word had spread

that a doctor was coming on a house call, and when I arrived the yard was full of neighbors. I became a little uncomfortable, as you can imagine—a white doctor coming to the slums to see a patient, surrounded by people watching me intently as I walked up to the door, which was open. I looked through the screen door at a living room full of people. I knocked, and one of the patient's daughters approached with a big grin. "You must be Dr. Smith."

"Yes, Ma'am," I answered, my voice cracking. She quickly ushered me in and gave me a hug. "We just so much appreciate you coming to see Momma. Come on in, and I'll take you to the back."

She took me through the small house to a back bedroom. Her mother was propped up in bed, an extremely old little black lady with snow-white hair, surrounded by grandchildren and great-grandchildren; they were all over her bed and scattered around the room. She gently spoke to them: "OK, ya'll kids, Granny loves you very much. This is my doctor. He's gonna take a look at me. Ya'll run along and play now."

Every last one of them kissed her on the cheek, told her they loved her, and left the room as they were told. She then grabbed my hand and patted it. "God bless you. He sent you to take care of me."

This patient had been running a fever, and she looked

much run-down. I examined her and concluded that she had pneumonia. I explained everything to her and told her I thought we should admit her to the hospital, for intravenous antibiotics. She said she'd do whatever I thought best. I made her a direct admit to the hospital, and called in orders. I told her I would see her in the morning. She patted my hand again and thanked me for the "special" treatment.

As I was leaving, another daughter asked me to come into the kitchen, where there was a buffet spread like I had only seen at my own grandmother's house, years before. She said, "We thought you might be hungry, so we made you a plate." They made a place for me at the table, and they fed me dinner; it was great—they made me feel like a king. The family took the woman to the hospital, and she did very well. My partner in charge of her care told me the family asks about me on every visit and tells her that they pray for me every day. They might be the only thing that's keeping me here on this earth.

On house calls like that, I learned the essence of what it must have felt like to be an old country doctor back in the day, and I have had very few things in my career that gave me as much professional satisfaction as taking care of that little old black lady in the slums. I knew then that I was doing exactly what I was meant to do.

So, while I might not be around to give advice to every young doctor who graduates from medical school, I'll just impart that advice now and hope someone reads it: Be a legend—make a house call.

Post Hoc

I have shared this house call story with medical students, interns, residents, and fellows I have known over the years. So many people go into medicine for reasons other than why they should—that is, to take care of people. At various times in my career I didn't take care of people as well as I should have … some days you just don't feel like it, you know? But every time I have had one of those days, I remember this story and it all becomes crystal clear to me. This is why I am here, and this is what I was meant to do.

"Taking care of people" can mean all kinds of things, when you think about it. There have been days when the *very best thing* I did that day was to get a patient a drink of water. Even the simplest acts of kindness take care of people. So what is the greater good? Is it Michael DeBakey, M.D., opening up a blocked coronary artery with a bypass, relieving angina pain, or could it be giving a dying patient a drink of water, a hand to hold, or just someone to sit beside them?

I know what most people would say...but I might disagree. Who is to say?

I think it is important for all physicians to recognize the extreme privilege with which they are entrusted: to take care of people. It is an opportunity. When someone asks a higher power for courage, strength, patience, or the ability to care for another, is he given courage, strength, patience, or the ability to care for another? Or simply given the opportunity to serve others?

I now realize that this house call was more for me and my benefit than it was for my patient.

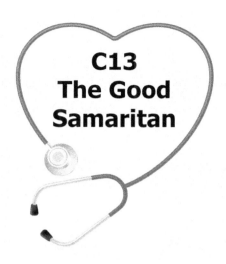

C13
The Good Samaritan

It had been a particularly bad call weekend; I honestly cannot remember exactly how long I had been awake. Just one of those weekends when everyone was sick and all of the patients seemed as if they were the most complicated patients one could have to care for ... a weekend when every single page spelled impending disaster, and another three hours without sleep. A weekend from hell itself—and just when I thought it couldn't get any worse, it definitely could.

After working from early Sunday morning, about 3 a.m, till 8 p.m. that night, I decided to check the ER for any of our patients—an effort to save myself the frustration of leaving only to get called back. Predictably, we had two patients there: one patient was critically ill; the other, Mr. Williams, was less ill but had problems breathing from his long history of smoking. I had seen him many times. I ordered an arterial blood-gas measurement, a chest X-ray, and some breathing medicine. I then quickly went about the business of stabilizing the more critically ill patient. When we were ready to take the critical patient to the ICU, I asked the nurse to call me when the lab and X-rays were completed on Mr. Williams, and told her I would come back to make a disposition with him. I hurried upstairs to continue my work on the extremely critical patient.

The ER nurse called me a couple of hours later, about 11 p.m., and told me that Mr. Williams' studies were back. When I arrived back in the emergency room, Mr. Williams was sleeping quietly. The results of his arterial blood-gas study prior to receiving his breathing treatment were really pretty good, for him. The chest X-ray was clear. I went into his room and woke him.

"Mr. Williams, looks like everything checks out OK. I'm going to let you go home. Do you need a prescription for your medicines?"

He looked disappointed. "You aren't going to put me in the hospital?"

"No sir, I'm not. Your ABG's are actually better than they usually are, and I see no evidence of pneumonia. The cigarettes are killing you. If you would just take your medicine and at least cut back on your smoking, I think you would breathe a lot easier."

"Well, if you ain't gonna keep me, you need to get me some oxygen to use at home." "Mr. Williams, I can't do that either. Your ABG's show that you don't need it and Medicare will not pay for it if you do not meet criteria. And I know you can't afford to simply buy everything yourself, not to mention the fact that I just don't think it's the right thing. The right thing is for you to take your medicines and cut back on your smoking."

He was clearly frustrated over this little lecture and made it known by saying, "You're a QUACK!"

"I may be a quack, but I'm *your* quack tonight, and I'm taking care of you based on sound medical principles and judgment. I'm sorry you feel that way." With that, I left the room, signed the discharge order, and went back to the ICU to continue stabilization of the critically ill patient.

I was up all night with the ICU patient—placing lines, adjusting medicines to maintain blood pressure, starting a slow continuous form of dialysis, and getting ventilator settings correct. At about 5 a.m. Monday morning, it finally seemed safe for me to leave the patient's bedside. I had gotten about four hours of sleep in a forty-eight-hour period, and the more I thought about it, the more rundown I felt. I decided to go home, power nap for a couple of hours, shower, and head back to the hospital.

I was parked in the ER dock parking area. As I walked through the ER, a fire-department ambulance was bringing Mr. Williams back to the emergency room. I just hung my head, sure that God was trying to kill me. I followed the ambulance gurney back inside to Room 5, the exact one he had been in just a few hours before. One of the paramedics told me they had transported him three times since 8 p.m. the night before; this was the second time to my hospital. They told me he had requested the county hospital when they transported him at 2 a.m. He was subsequently discharged.

But he seemed bound and determined to get admitted somewhere, and now here he was again on my doorstep. I re-examined him, ordered another arterial blood gas and a breathing treatment. This time, his ABG's were much better than when I had seen him a few hours before. Turns out the county hospital had also refused to write a prescription for any home oxygen or to admit him. I gave him just a brief lecture and discharged him to home.

It was about 6 a.m. at this point, and I had received a call from the ICU nurse; they were having an issue with the critical patient, so I went back upstairs to the unit and made some adjustments on my patient. At 7 a.m., I called my partner and told her what had happened. She agreed to cover me till noon so I could get a few hours of sleep.

As I was leaving the ER dock area, I saw Mr. Williams sitting on a bench outside. I had to walk right past him to get to my truck. We made eye contact. I said, "You need to get home and get some rest, Mr. Williams."

"I know, but I don't have a ride, and no one to come get me."

I stood there for a second, shaking my head. "Come on. I'll take you home."

"Would you, Doc? That would be great! I really appreciate it … and I'm sorry I called you a quack."

"It's OK, I've been called much worse. Just get in."

We left the hospital grounds, and I asked him for directions. He gave me a few streets to turn on but he clearly did not know where he lived. We passed a 7-Eleven convenience store and he said, "I know that place. I buy my cigarettes there."

"Mr. Williams, all 7-Elevens look alike, and there about five of them in this neighborhood alone." I knew he was completely clueless about where he lived. I called the ER and had them look up his address.

While we waited, he said, "Man, I sure am hungry and

could use a cup of coffee."

"What the hell," I said. "Me, too. What do you want? I'll go get it."

He gave me an extensive order of breakfast sandwiches and coffee; I went in and bought us breakfast, and we ate in the car while we waited on the ER to phone me his address. Once I got it, I drove him to his house, and there were four cars in his driveway. Turns out, no one paid any attention to him, and they had refused to come get him.

I saw Mr. Williams only twice after that day—once in the ER again, this time with burns to his upper lip and nostrils, as someone had given him that home oxygen he so desperately wanted; he just didn't know he wasn't supposed to light up around pure oxygen—something they forgot to tell him.

The second time was in the obituaries. Some people you just can't save.

So, my feeble attempt at being a Good Samaritan ended up with a lost little old man, a cup of hot coffee, and a shared breakfast for two in the front seat of my truck. Maybe that breakfast bought me a spot in heaven, but probably not.

Post Hoc

I suppose if there was another patient-care defining moment

for me, this would be it—but I was *so put out* with this guy. I know now he probably just wanted the attention and maybe someone to hang out with. It is so frustrating to try to take care of someone who will not pay any attention to what you say. Yet, all too often, that can be the majority of a physician's day in practice.

Clearly, there are some ignorant people who, for whatever reasons, refuse to assume responsibility for themselves. But I wonder if we shouldn't take a little time to find out why. More than once I have gone through this exercise and found the patient to be clinically depressed. I have found some who have been angry—angry at God, at their family, or at me. Sometimes people lose the will to live, and I believe that to be separate from being depressed. Finally, there comes a time for most chronically ill patients when they simply have had enough.

My internal-medicine program director, Jack Barnett, M.D., always said that part of being a good doctor is learning how to orchestrate a good death—very insightful and true words. I wonder sometimes how Dr. B would have handled Mr. Williams.

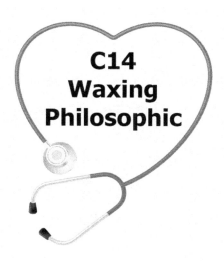

C14 Waxing Philosophic

Ron White, Larry the Cable Guy, George Carlin, and others have made a living simply pointing out the obvious to audiences worldwide. These guys have the ability to see an everyday situation in all of its absurdity and make it look totally ridiculous—and it is usually just that.

I have a very different way of looking at things, especially as they relate to people's actions. Quite frankly, these days little shocks me. I suspect that comes from seeing people at their very worst—people can really get themselves into a lot of trouble. Some would call my outlook cynical, others would say I am realistic, and still others would just call me an asshole and go about their business.

Although we sometimes think that we have the ability to change a person, a situation, or another person's view of a situation, we are just fooling ourselves. We do not have that kind of power. We cannot alter the subjective reality of another person. Trying to do so is an exercise in futility. After all, what someone *thinks* can be wrong ... but how they *feel* can never be wrong—a simple concept that is totally misunderstood by the majority of the population.

People take various courses in their lives, influenced by many things. The influences change as one gets older, yet the basic underlying construct of who a person really is, deep inside, remains. Why do people do this or that at certain points in their lives? Who really knows, as one can catch only a glimpse of another's heart? I would submit that a person's value system—the moral and ethical construct—predisposes that person to taking certain paths which can be altered by external influences. A crook can hang with a really good crowd and keep those criminal tendencies at bay, yet they are still there—only to rear their heads at unpredictable times. Remember the Enron debacle? I think it can also work in reverse. A really good person can hang with a bad element, and that's how good people get into bad situations. In the end, decisions are made, and bad decisions can be forgiven, but consequences remain. I can choose to smoke two packs of cigarettes for fifty years and ask forgiveness for destroying my lungs and blood vessels and spending a lot of money. And yes, I can be forgiven for that, but my lung cancer remains as a consequence of my choice.

No, people, you really can't fix stupid. You would think that, taking the Darwinian approach, stupid should have bred itself out of the population, but, for many reasons, it has not—and not just because there is always someone out there who will breed with anything and everything. It's much more complex than that. Education cannot, in and of itself, take care of the problem. I know some of the most brilliantly educated people—I wish I had only a thimbleful of their intelligence—yet most of them do not have sense enough to pour piss out of a boot. Sad, but so true.

The following call-night stories taught me a few lessons about myself and about people.

Mr. Coker was well into his eighties, a stroke victim who was bed bound, stiff as a board. He had a bevy of the usual medical problems. The nursing home sent him to the hospital for admission due to rectal bleeding. I was the unfortunate one on call for the group. The nurse working with me that night was my good friend Tommy Hughes, the Vietnam veteran, who was a dead ringer for Jerry Garcia of the Grateful Dead. (You remember him form a previous story in this book…love that guy!) We entered the room to start an IV, draw blood, and examine Mr. Coker. He was awake but did not talk or even acknowledge our presence. Tommy and I were having a conversation about whether the new radiation tech's breasts were augmented or her own—I don't think we ever found out—while Mr. Coker just passively endured the abdominal exam without saying a word.

Well, since he did present with rectal bleeding, I was obligated to confirm or deny the presence of that little problem, so I had to perform a rectal exam. Now I have to tell you: truly I would rather *get* a pap smear than have to perform a rectal exam, and I'm a guy! Nonetheless, I told Tommy, "Hey…let's roll him and let me check his butt for blood."

I gloved my hands, lubed up a finger, and did the digital rectal thing on poor Mr. Coker. When I put my finger in his rectum to check for blood, he spoke for the first time in the lowest, deadpan monotone voice: "Dammit … are ya fuckin' me?"

I was so embarrassed! My finger came out that man's butt quicker than a cat could lick its own. "Mr. Coker. I am so sorry. I didn't think you were aware of anything we were doing." He never said anything more. There was no blood in the rectum, by the way.

Tommy and I left the room stifling uncontrollable laughter. Finally, after I calmed down, I wondered. Why would that old man say something like that? It also made me wonder what was happening to him at the nursing home. I asked the social worker to look into things, and a few weeks later, an attendant was arrested for sexually abusing a number of residents. I learned a couple of very important things: NEVER assume. NEVER assume someone is not aware of what is happening. LISTEN to old people; they are not fools.

I sometimes marvel at the ignorance manifested in people's daily lives and attempt to find some means of justification. Sometimes the ignorance is understandable, but other times, I cannot discern a clue. The understandable circumstances of ignorance occur when someone is not educated enough to know better—for example, a patient doing something he didn't know was harmful, or my independent daughter saying or doing something that she has not been told specifically NOT to do. Far more difficult to understand, and much funnier, are circumstances when ignorance rears its head in the educated person, or the person who *really should know better.*

After one weekend of brutal call nights, one of my partners looked at me on Monday morning and asked, "How was you weekend? Mine was restful and good."

Oh yeah? "Have a look at me, and tell me what kind of

weekend you think I had! How about those bags and dark circles under my eyes. And the smell, since I haven't showered in twenty-four hours."

"Sorry I asked…"

Hopefully he won't make that mistake again.

Most of the hospitals I cover on call have active training and teaching programs. For the most part, I enjoyed the interaction, but some call nights you're just not in the mood. One night I was asked to see a patient for a group of residents, M.D.s in training, they couldn't figure out a couple of things. They told me the patient was lethargic and had slurred speech. When I saw the patient, I quickly realized they had been killing the poor little guy slowly over the previous three days, and he was dry as a chip. After curbing my desire to call the police to report a murder in progress, I called the sweet little beauty-queen resident M.D. and tried very nicely to explain the gross malpractice error occurring with this patient. She argued with me —but hey, if you don't want my opinion, don't fucking ask.

I told her that the patient she thought had "slurred speech" was, in fact, unable to talk because his mouth was so dry from being fluid-deprived that his tongue was stuck in the roof of his mouth. In reality, he was saying only two things: "Get me a drink of water," and, "Get me a Doctor." *Sports Il-*

lustrated Swim Suit Model, M.D., did not appreciate my dry humor, but then again, I didn't appreciate her ignorance and failure to acknowledge it. I told her it was one thing to want to be a doctor, but that sometimes you have to actually pay attention to what's going on—kids these days. She gave me the obligatory "Fuck you!" stare and walked off. She will soon learn the ropes just as I did, or she'll be history.

One special night on call, a patient of ours came to the hospital but had no chief complaint listed. A male patient with no complaint given—well, that could only mean one thing: venereal disease. Guys, for some reason, are embarrassed to tell the nurses they have the "drip." I guess they want to keep "the door open" in case the nurse wants a little exam-room action. Fully prepared for this, I went back to examine the patient. He was a portly, young Hispanic man who looked to be in good health.

I asked him what was wrong. "I think I'm infected," he said. I asked him to drop his shorts to examine his private parts. They looked OK to me, so I asked him, "What make you think you have an infection? Have you been burning when you pee or had a drip?"

With a troubled look on his face, he answered politely, "No, sir." I asked, "Did the girl you were with tell you she was infected?" Now, as we have discussed, not much catches me off guard, but I must admit his answer blew me away. As he bowed his head, he said, "I wasn't with a girl."

"OK, did the guy you were with say anything?"

"Hey man, I ain't no queer!"

"Easy man, sorry! But help me out here, you weren't with a girl or a guy … who or what were you with?"

He said, "I went inside a momma pig."

I struggled to understand. "Do you mean you had sexual intercourse with a fat chick?"

"No sir, I mean a momma pig."

"A sow?"

"Yes, sir." I said OK, and excused myself for a moment—to collect myself and my thoughts, and to laugh my ass off.

I thought long and hard about what to do. There were no specific venereal pathogenic organisms I knew of that required a pig vector. I decided to have a little bit of fun. I told a couple of the "cool" nurses to listen to the room speaker. I gathered up a toy "tricorder" —you Trekkies will remember the one Bones used to carry. That's right, the thing that could diagnose and fix every ailment known to modern medicine. I turned on the in-room speaker and went back into the room. I asked the patient to recount all that he had told me; just to make sure I had everything right, and he complied. He asked me what the instrument was, and I told him it was a "pig penis scanner" and it would tell me if there was any infection. He bought it, and I beeped that thing all around his perineum. "OK, you're clean. But NEVER have sex with another pig, OK?"

"Oh, yes, sir, I promise—and thanks, man."

"No problem, wait here for your discharge instructions."

When I returned to the nurse's station, they were in tears, as was I. I finished writing up the chart, replete with the discharge instructions, "DON'T BANG ANY MORE PIGS." Got in trouble for that one from medical records, but what the hell. It was a once-in-a-lifetime chance.

I try not to be philosophical on call nights anymore. Certain things just simply are not logical.

Post Hoc

I have gotten a lot of mileage out of the "sex with a momma pig" story over the years. I still just shake my head in amazement. What possesses some of these people? I know; it's futile to try to understand. But it's a bad habit for me: attempting to reach an understanding and fanning a philosophy about things that happen. Still, there are some situations where that task is just not possible.

People do some really stupid things and, believe me, I

have seen most of them. They place various things in places where they are not designed to be placed. They drink things that are not supposed to be drunk. They eat things that are not supposed to be eaten. And they take drugs they shouldn't be taking. The strangest thing is that even when people are caught red-handed in these various exploits, they will lie, feign innocence, or blame-shift such that none of it is really *their* fault. Only rarely will someone in a stupid predicament come absolutely clean with the truth about how they got there. And sometimes you just wish they wouldn't.

During my years in medicine, I have simply come to the realization that whatever predicament a patient finds himself in, it matters not. Whatever it is has happened or is stuck, and however it happened or however it got stuck or whatever the warped thought process of the person involved, the collective "we" in medicine must deal with it anyway. Still, like a car accident, where you know you shouldn't really look but you just can't help it, sometimes I just can't help myself. I ask, and most of the time I wish I hadn't.

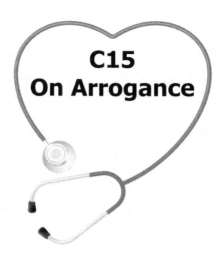

C15
On Arrogance

I never cease to be amazed at the opinion some people have of themselves and the arrogant actions that spring from that mindset. I know all of the deep psychological differential diagnoses and reasons why some people adopt this type of attitude and behavior. Although frankly, I think these psychological excuses are made as an attempt at resolution by weak-minded individuals to justify being treated like shit by complete and utter assholes. Arrogant people are just bullies, and they behave like children—SPOILED children at that. The best way to deal with them comes straight from the Bible.

Now please do not get me wrong. I am no theologian or

biblical scholar—hell, I'm not even a decent Catholic—but I do remember the concept of "spare not the rod," or something like that. Honestly, I think these people should be treated in the only fashion that speaks to a bully: You hit them as hard as you can, right in the mouth … perhaps not necessarily in the literal sense, but certainly in the figurative one. It's the only effective means of dealing with them. Our problem? We enable their behavior.

My son is an elite gymnast. He trains in a world-class gym. The other gymnasts who train there are excellent, as well. I have learned that, to be a good gymnast, one must not only be an excellent technician, but also must have a certain swagger—an air of cockiness, if you will. They have to possess the confidence to go out and nail an exercise and also to kick the asses of anyone who tries to do it better then they can. My son is like that, in a way, but in a much kinder and gentler fashion, if that is possible.

There is a boy on his team; we'll call him Satan. Satan torments my son—he is a bully in the strictest sense. My son complains bitterly about Satan to the point of wanting to quit. When he asked my advice, I told him, "You grab Satan by the ears. You tell him not to hit you or push you anymore. Tell him if he does, you are going to hit him as hard as you can right in the mouth."

"But Dad," my gentle son answers. "I don't know if I can do that. I'm just not that kind of person."

"If you really want Satan to leave you alone, you will do what I say."

A few days later, my son showed me a bruise he had on his arm where Satan had hit him. "Why did you let him hit you?" I cried, all the while getting ready to head to the gym and beat the ever-loving shit out of Satan's father, mother, brother, the coach, and anyone else who might look at me the wrong way.

Then my son says: "That was before I hit him back and knocked him down." Excuse me while I BEAM a bit. As I was feeling quite proud of the boy, he said, "But Daddy, I'm still really not that kind of person."

Kind of a poignant statement, wouldn't you agree? Stopped me in my tracks.

Some of the most arrogant people I know are physicians and, in a lot of circumstances, I very much dislike dealing with them. Most of their arrogance is in passive-aggressive form. It is one of the reasons I really do not like to hang out with doctors, for the most part. And arrogant bully physicians are especially annoying on call nights.

One particular call night I had to deal with my own personal bully, a surgeon. We'll call him Satan, M.D. I will not go into details—just suffice it to say that the man is the most arrogant asshole I have ever come across in all my years of practicing medicine, and that speaks volumes. There is a colloquialism I have personally coined during my career: "If you're going to be a prick, you better be a smart one and be able to back it up." There is really no place for a stupid prick, yet that's what we have in Satan, M.D. He carries a highly inflated opinion of himself, his expertise, and his intelligence. The reason I know this? He opens his mouth. Smart people stay quiet; they know when they're right and they're secure in that fact regardless of what another might think. Satan, M.D., opens his mouth and proves his ignorance. The truth is, Satan, M.D., is not a very good doctor.

A confrontation between the two of us occurred one night, handled the only way he knows how: by voice mail on my office phone. How courageous. I was so angry at this guy for a lot of reasons, not least the fact that he wouldn't return my calls. I wanted to march over to the hospital, run this guy down, and beat the crap out of him. But a part of me remained intimidated for some reason.

And then I remembered what my son had said: "I'm not that kind of person." Hmmm. You know what? I am really not that kind of person, either. But the only way to deal with your bullies is to stand up to them, knock the shit out of them, and then stand there and look at them with *this* look on your face: "You DON'T want anymore of this."

So that is what I did, in a figurative sense. Since Satan, M.D., wouldn't return my calls, I sent him a certified letter—which I guess could be considered as chicken shit as his actions. Anyway, in it, I told him I didn't like what he did, that it would be the last time he did it to me, that I would not tolerate it anymore, and that if it ever happened again, there would, I promised, be unpleasant consequences. I was still so pissed off at him I almost hoped that he'd try some of his lame bullshit again. Now don't misunderstand me; I'm not a warmonger or anything like that. I have had my ass whipped a few times, but *nobody ever enjoyed doing it,* and I promise he won't, either. I didn't know if "hitting him in the mouth," either physically or figuratively, would realistically accomplish anything. I'm not that naïve. But I sure felt better.

As I have explained to you multiple times, and at the risk of being quite redundant, the most fragile thing in the world is not the finest glass, porcelain, crystal, or china; as I have told you; it is a doctor's ego. I am going to have to include myself in that discussion, but I do try and keep that in check.

Arrogant people have a disconnect. Some have a delusion disorder where they actually believe they are better than others. Some use arrogance as a mask, a cover, a defense mechanism to hide their deep-seated insecurities—things they've never dealt with or issues they simply do not have the psychological wherewithal to confront. I think the latter explanation would include the majority of these people.

Dealing with some doctors on call nights is like dealing with one's grade-school bully. So the question remains: How do you deal with an arrogant person? I believe you "hit them in the mouth." It's the only thing they understand. And like my son, every time I have had to do it, I realize I am not really that kind of person either.

Post Hoc

As I look back and read this story, I realize I have softened a bit. While that physician and his actions still make me angry, I think I rather feel quite sorry for him. Satan, M.D., has not changed over the years. I almost did not include this story, but I believe it has some relevance for new doctors, those wanting to become doctors, and, really, anyone else who must deal with difficult people in relationships or business.

Dealing with difficult people is a fact of life; we all must do it at one point or another. I know everyone has their own way of doing so. I believe that to deal effectively with these jerks, one must give them clear boundaries. And they need to understand that whenever they cross these boundaries, there'll be consequences. At the very least a face-to-face talk, devoid of emotion, and simply stating facts. There is no room for emotional, intellectual, or physical domination in any relationship. When boundaries are crossed, the person who crosses them needs to be told that will not be accepted or tolerated.

For new doctors or those thinking of becoming doctors, please remember that doctors' egos are the most fragile thing in the whole world, and we typically do not take criticism well. But there are ways to get along with most everyone, and ways to make your point in a nonthreatening way—and this is always in the best interest of patient care. Still, there will be times when a colleague will get ugly about something; just count on it. And when it happens, it often becomes personal. Do me and you a favor. Do not handle things as I have done in certain circumstances, as I did in the story. Take the high road. It will be in your best interest and that of your patient.

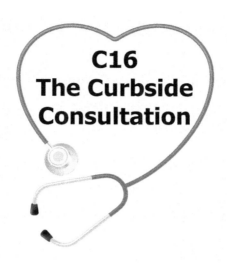

C16
The Curbside Consultation

We all know people who, regardless of their station in life, will always try to get something for nothing. The situation is no different when it comes to dealing with other physicians on call nights. I mean, it would be one thing if these people would just preface their conversations with, "I don't want you to get paid for this, but I need an opinion on what to do." And these types of physician calls come at all hours, day and night.

The classic example is the early-morning call from an ER doctor explaining a clinical situation that he or she is just "not comfortable" about. Here's what he or she is really saying: "I need you to assume some liability with me for the care of this patient, in case I make a mistake." Predictably, your name will be placed in big, bold letters prominently on the front of the record. "Discussed with Dr. Smith. He agrees with the plan." In many circumstances the patient you are being "curb-sided" about is not even someone you've ever placed your hands upon. I think that most ER physicians believe that writing another physician's name on the record somehow excuses some of their own liability. How naive.

Every sub-specialist I know has fallen victim to the infamous curbside consultation while making rounds in the hospital. It usually starts with seeing a doctor you know. Pleasantries are exchanged. This small talk—mental medical foreplay—proceeds. "How is your golf game?" "How is your hospital service?" "Did you see all of the cuts in reimbursement this month?" And on and on.

After these exchanges, a word is uttered that lets you know you have fallen victim. And that word is, "Hey ..." Now, on the surface you might think that this is a benign word, but to those of us who render hospital opinions for a living, it invokes a series of responses, which include, but aren't limited to, rolling the eyes, a sick feeling in the stomach, bitter contempt for a lazy colleague who doesn't want to be bothered with something they might actually have to think about, a case of heartburn, and loss of appetite. This is quite different from when a colleague calls in a situation where they really need help—those situations are easy to ascertain, the one thing that really excites most sub-specialists I know, and, frankly, the reason we actually still like this business.

In one hospital I've worked in, a certain internist has a reputation far and wide as the master of the curbside consultation. He is an absolute *wizard*. I have seen him do three at once for the same patient. He knows all the tricks. Over the years I have discovered that if he doesn't see you, he generally will not consult you, so the most experienced of us remember the stealth lessons we all learned as interns or residents.

It is a carefully scripted dance he performs, which goes something like this: you will generally spot him from down the hall—lab coat open, collared shirt unbuttoned to the nipple line, exposing a massively hairy chest, a prominent golden Star of David amulet hanging from his neck.

"How are you doing today, Kyle?" he'll call out.

"Oh, hi, Mike. Good, how about you?"

"I was doing OK till I just read that damn Medicare bulletin. Do you know what they are trying to do to us now? They are cutting us across the board. How do you think we will be able to earn a living anymore?"

"Jeez, I don't know, Mike. Just gets worse every year."

"Yeah. It pisses me off. Big business is all into medicine, raping us all, making big bucks off us and leaving us to do all of the work. It's that damn Clinton, you know."

"Yeah … Well, you try to have a good day. Stay out of the poorhouse, OK?"

As you are walking away, thinking you've escaped, you hear THAT word, and you utter another word—"SHIT!"—to yourself.

"Hey!"

"Yeah, Mike, were you calling me?" Of course, you know he did.

"Yeah … hey, listen. I've got this little lady they did a CT scan on the other day and her kidney function is going down. What do you think?"

"Well, Mike, I don't really know. Did she get a contrast study? Is she on any medicine that would cause her kidney function to go down? Are you sure she's obstructed for any reason? Do you think she may be a little on the dry side?"

As he intently listens to your differential diagnosis, he nods incessantly and says,

"You know, I just am not certain."

"Well, I think I would check all of that out, do a renal ultrasound, check urinary electrolytes and urinary eosinophils, and check her medicines. Because, you know, when they develop kidney trouble in the hospital, it is usually something we did to them."

He nods in understanding.

You continue: "Do you want me to take a look at the patient?"

Which, translated, means: "Hey, you fat bastard, I just did the whole consult for you. And now you're going to get the money and the glory for being such a dumb ass."

And he always replies, "No, I know you're busy. I'll just handle it myself."

After feeling generally intellectually molested, you move on about your rounds, having learned once again. It pays to remain stealthy.

The dreaded curbside consult probably does serve a purpose for most physicians; you learn a little here and there. But for some, like my colleague Mike, it's just a classic example of getting something for nothing. I just figure if Medicare and private insurance ever go to a system where the primary physician is responsible for paying for all of these consultations, I may have to go back to digging ditches.

Post Hoc

You know, after all these years, I still love Mike (not his real name) to death, but he still pisses me off. And he is just one extreme on the spectrum. I didn't tell you about the other end of the spectrum in the original story, but now I feel compelled.

There are doctors who obtain medical consultations on their patients for no clear cut reason, other than shared liability for malpractice, and for EVERYTHING remotely possible, even the most simple and mundane abnormality or even sometimes when there *is* no abnormality… and these physicians do not have the common courtesy to simply call and ask your opinion. Usually this type of consultation practice is done by the younger doctors who don't know better or the older doctors who have always done it that way. I don't know why they do this; I would never do that to a colleague. I have always felt that I should give the person respect enough to call, review the case, and tell her what I am worried about and why I want or need the opinion. In most circumstances, it saves them a lot of legwork in the chart by focusing on the problem, and they appreciate it.

I must also mention the "new breed" of doctors, the specialty of the "me" generation: the "hospitalist." These are typically young internal medicine doctors who shun private practice, enjoy shift work, are raising a family and want to choose their hours, or are simply hanging around waiting to get into a particular fellowship. Some of these young doctors are quite good, and some are frankly lazy. The lazy ones are the ones who will consult every sub-specialty in internal medicine on each and every case—maybe it's insecurity in some circumstances, but I think it's sheer laziness in most. And I am not talking about those cases where patients are critically ill with multi-system failure; consults are always appropriate and needed there.

I would hope that some day, there will be a special-qualification board examination to practice as a hospitalist. I think these physicians can do a lot of good, but there should be some standards or guidelines; that's all I am saying.

Having said all of this, I never turn down the opportunity to help, even the laziest of my colleagues.

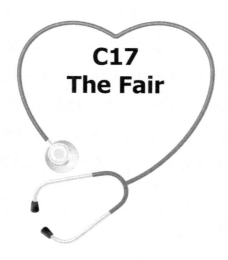

C17
The Fair

The State Fair of Texas is a time honored ritual occurring every October in Dallas. Adults and children, alike, have looked forward to the Fair for decades. Exhibits, stock shows, Midway rides, and games...and side shows to include bearded ladies, dwarfs, Siamese twins, the World's smallest horse. the World's longest snake, or the World's largest dog, just to name a few of the side shows featured over the years. In recent years, the food items have been a tremendous draw... fried Twinkies, fried Oreos, and even fried butter. Why anyone would want to eat fried butter is beyond me, but they do. Of course, there are the age old favorites at the Fair...Fletchers Corny Dogs and Belgian Waffles. No Fair visit is complete without them.

I can remember almost every Fair season from the time I was a school boy. The school district would allow one day for all the students to be out of school and would give them a free ticket and bus token to go to the Fair. Mom and Dad would fork over $5-$10 for a day of rides, food, and souvenirs. And you HAD to buy the souvenirs...we ALL knew those Midway games were rigged and you really would never walk out of there with a stuffed animal larger than you were. It was an ALL day affair.

Sometimes Mom would take us, sometimes Dad would take us, and sometimes they both would. As we got a little older, we were allowed to go by ourselves back in those days. Mom pretty much like watching our escapades on the rides, with the games, and taking in the corny dog culinary delight. Except for the occasional exhibit that would interest Dad, you could tell he just took us because we wanted to go... well, that, and they did serve cold draft beer, which I am sure made it more palatable. It didn't really matter, though...we were just glad he was there...and we were glad when Mom was there too.

I suppose, as I look back on it, it was a time when no one had a lot of money and the State Fair afforded some great cheap fun for everyone. I have a lot of good memories from the State Fair of Texas...memories of a much simpler time, a time for family, and a time for friends.

As I grew older, I got too busy to ever go to the State Fair. School was always in full swing and it just seemed that I never could carve out the time to go...and I lost interest, not wanting to fight the crowds. And this continued from the time I was in college, medical school, graduate school, internship, residency, fellowship, and private practice.

After entering private practice, my first practice partner was also my senior most partner, Steven Rinner, MD. One of the brightest and most gifted physicians I have ever had the pleasure of learning from. I loved him then, as I do to this day...he remains the only one I have ever found to actually match my sarcasm. We actually had fun working together, trading sarcastic patient stories...I even can remember him laughing out loud a few times!! Steve was and is a revered physician...I learned important lessons from him, not limited to, but including a professional work ethic, the ability to tell someone exactly what you think, for better or worse, and how to be a constant student of medicine. It was especially nice because we lived in the same little community outside of Dallas...checking up on the other after weekend on call was really cool, because he would come over to my house, or I would head over to his house and we would sit and talk about the patients for the following week.

Steve and I worked long hours, to be sure. We helped each other too, such that if I finished my work, I would not go home until Steve had finished too...if I had to pitch in and help him, that's just what I would do. And he would do the same for me. Nobody went home until all the work was done.

During the workday a number of years past, we were sitting across from one another in a nurses station writing our notes. He said, "Hey...you take off tomorrow afternoon and take your kids to the Fair. It's Rockwall Fair Day. The kids are out of school." Of course, so wrapped up in work, I didn't even know...certainly no one at home mentioned it. I said, "Awww...that's OK...I'll stay and work...the service is too big. Besides, I don't even think they WANT to go." He just stopped writing his notes and gave me the stare..."Take your kids to the Fair..." I could tell he really meant that statement. I meekly replied, "OK".

I took the kids to the Fair and, much like my Dad, just hung around, gave them cash to waste on the mundane rides, games, and junk food...all while I was able to enjoy cold draft beer. I was glad I took them after I did, although I hate to say I did it begrudgingly. We did it another couple of years, until they got tired of me and wanted to hang with their friends.

But they still talk about going to the Fair, after all these years. I still never really quite grasped why Steve would be so adamant about me taking off an afternoon to take my kids to the Fair.

Medicine, in all of its glory, is truly a harlot of magnificent proportion. She will rob the very essence of humanity from you. She takes so much precious time and can sometimes be so selfish, not allowing you even one moment to yourself, let alone to those whom you love. Sometimes you have to stand up and confront the harlot...and say enough is enough. That is a much harder proposition than it sounds.

You see, it isn't about the things we do with those whom we love...it is about the time we spend with them. Too often in medicine, this is a hard lesson to learn. Steve knew this... I had no clue.

Many years later, I did further training and was part of initiating a new type of medical practice which merged with our existing practice. I was all caught up in it. It was higher pressure, more surgically oriented, required more time, and more commitment. I became consumed with perfection of this new practice and consumed with making a name for myself. Things that should have been priority became secondary. I was spending less and less time at home...less and less time with my family. I reasoned that it was all right because I was providing for them...I was able to work and give them things I had been denied growing up.

After a failed marriage, I was determined to be a really good single father. I continued to think that being a really good father meant giving the children things I did not have growing up. After receiving these things, the kids were always very appreciative and were quick to say thank you and give me a big hug.

A short time later, one of my children started having problems with depression. Not to get into the clinical details and all of the issues surrounding this depression, because those are not related to the REAL issue and point I am trying to make. I made my own children feel like they were not important and not a priority. It was not because I did not love my children...it was not because I did not provide for my children...it was not because my intentions were not good. I neglected to realize the one thing that was needed of me...it was the very thing Steve knew and had learned...it was the thing I understood about my own father. It's simply the TIME. It's not the things...it's the time.

Now, why would I write a chapter in a book about medicine and tell everyone about my flaws as a father? It is because I am hoping that anyone who reads this book who might be considering a career in anything that requires so much of a person, will hear and understand...the most important and precious thing we can ever offer is our time.

For the new physician or for those who are studying to become physicians, if you have a family or are planning to in the future, please do not take this lightly. The best advice I can give you is the same advice that was given to me...don't be like me and focus on the least important things and make them more important than they really are. The future is in our children and our families.

So, take your kids to the Fair.

Post Hoc

I really do not have more to say about this...I have revisited it many times. One of the hardest lessons I have ever had to learn is the importance of simply giving time and being with those who matter to us most. In a profession that, at times, can truly be life and death, it is easy to perhaps gain a higher opinion of one's own self worth. I look back on my own experience...it makes me want to laugh...and cry at the same time. And I suppose the take home here is to never take yourself too seriously.

I am not a perfect man and even less of a perfect father. I love all of my children deeply, but I have short changed them...

it's simply the time. When you spend time, you tell them in no uncertain terms that they have importance and priority in your life. I've failed them in that at times. But thank God I realized it before it was too late.

I received a message from my ex-wife, as we have been dealing with a couple of child related issues. She simply said, "Good Daddy"...I replied back, "Not good...but better".

Honestly, take your kids to the Fair!

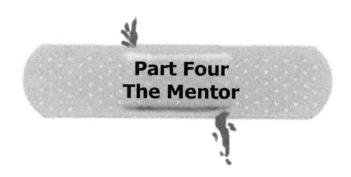

Part Four
The Mentor

This may be the single most important thing I have written or story I have told, the one that has had the most impact on me. My eyes well up with tears each and every time I read it. In medicine, we are taught to revere our professors; in this case, I loved mine.

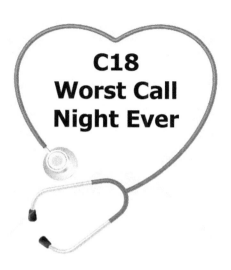

C18
Worst Call Night Ever

In the third year of medical school the doctor-to-be starts his or her clinical rotations, when time is spent in the hospital training in the various disciplines of medicine. This is an exciting time, because it really is the first glimpse at actually becoming a physician. And I particularly loved the fact that the teaching occurred on the hospital wards, discussing real-live patient problems in Socratic fashion at the feet of the attending doctor.

I met The Mentor when I was a third-year medical student, when I was completing my internal-medicine ward rotation. I was intimidated from the start. He was tall and lanky, of average build, and balding on the crown of his head, and he wore glasses. I thought he was brilliant—he just looked god awful smart. He was board certified in internal medicine, nephrology, and critical care medicine. The Mentor was actually *excited* about making rounds, and it showed in every bit of his being. He greeted doctors and nurses as he bounced down the halls, occasionally stopping to ask questions of those he knew well. "Hey, did you make the hockey game last night? Did you see that incredible play?"

We had a ritual when we arrived at the nurse's station. The medical students and interns would gather the charts of our patients, load them on a chart rack, and get a cup of coffee for everyone, including The Mentor … always one sugar, one cream. We then sat at a conference table and presented the new cases to The Mentor. He would listen intently, making mental notes of how someone had done this wrong or that wrong, but he never interrupted. After listening to each case, he would finish his coffee and say, "OK. Let's go see 'em." With that, we would head to the room of the patient. The Mentor had a habit of putting his arm around you and patting you on the back, especially when he knew you were wrong about something and he was getting ready to rip your ass.

He always entered the patient's room with a smile on his face, and made that patient feel as if he or she was the most important person in the world. He would talk with them and ALWAYS … and I do mean ALWAYS … take the patient's blood pressure himself. He insisted that we do the same. I understood in later years why, and it wasn't what I had suspected at the time; I always thought he did it because he didn't trust the nurse to get it right. That was partly correct, but even more, he did it because it initiated contact with the patient. A bond is formed when a doctor touches you, and no one understood that better than The Mentor.

After the examination, The Mentor would look at the entire chart and concentrate intently on the laboratory values. God help you if you did not have your patients' labs drawn at 4 a.m. just so the results would be posted on the chart by the time rounds started. The lab hated that about The Mentor. After looking at the lab work, he would proceed to pick apart this or that, and explain why what you did or why your thought processes were wrong. Then he would right the ship and give you some direction along with something to read so that you would not forget it. He had absolutely no problem telling you exactly what he thought. Occasionally you'd make an egregious mistake and he would come unglued, to the point of getting into your face with his classic statement, "What the hell were ya thinkin'?" followed up quickly with, "Well, looks like ya fucked the dog on this one."

After his tirade, it was done and over with, and The Mentor would always put his healing hand and arm around you, pat you on the back, and start your broken spirit on the road to mending. It was never personal with The Mentor; everything he did was for the good of the patient, and to make you a better doctor.

After that rotation, I admired The Mentor more than I could ever write or say. You always knew where you stood with him, and I wanted to be just like him.

Through the miracle of the intern and resident matching program, on "match day" I matched an internal medicine residency at the hospital where I had first met The Mentor. And as luck would have it, he was my attending on my very first rotation. I was ecstatic. I read incessantly and tried so hard to be a doctor that The Mentor would be proud to have trained. I started rounds two hours before he arrived to make sure I knew all I could about what had happened with the patients the night before, I looked at every X-Ray study we ordered, and I made damn sure I knew all of the labs or anything else he might be interested in knowing about any particular patient.

We made rounds twice a day on all of the patients, even though he would only get paid for one visit. He said that if someone was sick enough to be in the hospital, he or she deserved to be seen by his physician twice a day, so that is what we did. Sometimes it could be grueling, but we would never think of leaving until all of the work was done. He would never dump any work on the call person.

The Mentor made medicine fun, even though sometimes it really *wasn't* much fun. He had all kinds of quips and quotes, many of which he became famous for in the hospital. For example when we saw a patient who was effectively dehydrated, he would say, "Jesus! He's as dry as a popcorn fart!" Or if you happened to do some something really good, he would say something like, "Well, NOW you're fartin' through silk." He had countless other witticisms. Sometimes he could be a little scatterbrained, but that was only because he was always thinking ahead. He was adamant about certain things, and one of them was doing rectal exams for fecal occult blood on every patient admitted. He did this because most kidney patients have some element of anemia, and he wanted to make sure he didn't miss a case of anemia due to blood loss from the stomach or colon.

One day we had a number of new admissions to the service, some admitted by the on-call nephrologists. When we loaded up the chart rack, The Mentor always made sure we had developing cards to check the admitted patients' stools for occult blood. After each rectal exam, he closed the hem occult card and put it in his lab coat pocket. Then he said, in an excited tone of voice, "Hey, after rounds we'll get a coffee and do turd rounds." We'd sit to have coffee and write the notes and orders on the charts, and we systematically opened the cards and developed them to see if there was any sign of blood.

On one particular day, The Mentor forgot to write the names of the patients on the cards—and two of them were positive. "Dammit!" he said. "All right, guess what you need to do this afternoon while I go to the office." I simply said, "Yes sir, I do." I had to go do another rectal exam on each and every patient, to find the two who were positive. I wasn't a very popular resident with the patients that day.

The Mentor made me feel like a real doctor; he made me feel that I was important to him, and a necessary part of his team. And while he would be the very first to jump down your throat and take you to task, he was also the first to be right there in your corner and defend you. One evening before we left for the day, we admitted a very noncompliant young dialysis patient with fever and chills. The Mentor brought an extensive dialysis folder on her so that we would have everything we needed to know. She had lost a kidney transplant because she stopped taking her immunosuppressive medications, and she had been relegated to dialysis for a long time. She had man-eating high blood pressure and was on a ton of powerful medicine.

After The Mentor and I examined her, he had to leave to go catch a dialysis shift. "Hey," he asked. "Do you think you can write these [admission] orders for me? I gotta run catch that shift. I'm on call tonight anyway. Just double-check these medicines to make sure they are correct and that she's taking them, OK?"

"Yes, sir!" I was beaming because he trusted me to take care of that for him. I went back to the patient and went over all the medicines with her. She never made eye contact with me, just nodded after I asked about each medicine and the dosage listed. I wrote the orders as The Mentor had told me to do.

Later that evening, I received a call at home from a fellow resident. He was on call and had been called to the floor to clarify my orders because the blood-pressure medications were in large doses. He said her blood pressure was high, but he wasn't sure if the doses were correct. I told him to double-check with the patient and the dialysis note I had attached to the chart. Feeling a bit uneasy, now that one of my resident buddies was questioning the medicines, I asked him to call The Mentor, since he was on call, to confirm that giving her the medicine was OK. He checked the chart and the patient, and told the nurse it was all right to give the medicines as they had been ordered.

When I arrived early the next morning to start rounds before The Mentor arrived, I saw him in the ICU. He was obviously very tired, looking as if he'd been without sleep all night, and he was dressed in the clothes he had left the hospital in the night before. I asked him what had happened, and he told me the patient we admitted the night before had crashed on the floor due to extremely low blood pressure. She was intubated on a ventilator and was requiring massive doses of pressors (powerful medications to keep her blood pressure up).

One of the cardiologists was in the room doing an echocardiogram to see if there was any fluid around the heart. Going over her chart, I found that the blood cultures we had drawn the night before were all positive, meaning that she had bacteria growing in her bloodstream.

I was devastated. "Sir, I am so sorry," I told The Mentor. "I think I killed her." He gave me a look that I cannot describe, grabbed me by the arm, and hurried me into a conference room. In a very angry voice, he said, "You listen to me. I don't want to ever hear you say anything like that ever again! Do you understand me?"

"Yes, sir," I meekly replied.

He went on: "What happened to her was nobody's fault. If I thought for a second that you fucked up and caused this, I would have called you at home and had you drag your ass in here and help me take care of her. Don't ever say what you just said again." And with that, we went back to the patient's room.

The cardiologist was completing the echocardiogram. The Mentor asked, "What do you see, Kirk?" He answered, "There's no effusion, but she has the largest valve vegetation I believe I have ever seen."

"I thought so. Thanks for coming out early, man." The Mentor looked at me, never said anything, and then gave me a little punch in the chest. When he finished his note on the chart, he said, "I've gotta go do an early-morning shift. I'll be back in an hour. You keep going. Oh, and read my note—then tonight I want you to read about endocarditis and septic shock."

He had written in the chart that the patient was suffering from hypotension, multiple organ dysfunction, and septic shock caused by staphylococcal endocarditis with massive bacteremia.

During my three years of residency, I rotated with The Mentor six or seven times. He trusted me and on some nights he knew I was on call, he'd have me check something for him, especially when I became an upper-level resident. I'll never forget a conversation we had one evening when I was on second-year rotation. We had a very sick patient who required an emergent abdominal surgery. If something surgically particularly interested him, The Mentor would go into the OR and watch the surgery, something I learned from him and still do today. After the surgery this one night, we were changing clothes, and he started a conversation with me.

"Hey, I definitely think you would make a damn good nephrologist. What do you think about that? Do you have any interest in going further?" I told him I would be interested. I didn't want to tell him that I wanted to be just like him.

"OK," he said. "Then we need to start on your applications." He helped me get an application to the program he wanted me to attend, the same one he and so many of his partners had attended. I also applied to some of the other programs in the area.

I promptly received an interview to the "chosen" program. And I know why. I also interviewed at a couple of other places. I didn't hear anything for a while, but finally I got a letter from the University of Arkansas for Medical Sciences, offering me a job. I was ecstatic. I sought out The Mentor the next day and told him. The only thing he said was, "What the hell are you gonna do up there? Learn to dialyze a fucking pig? You just wait a while before you commit to anything." Shortly afterward, I received a call from the program director at the "chosen" program, offering me a job.

Due to a lot of things I will not bore you with, I decided to enter into the practice of emergency medicine instead of nephrology. I know I disappointed The Mentor and others. But they never once berated me over that move and, since I practiced at one of the large hospitals, I think I was a big help in taking care of their patients when they were on call. After seven years in the emergency room, I had had enough and started to look at private-practice opportunities. The Mentor and his group took me in. We practiced together, and they ultimately gave me the honor of buying into the practice. And now The Mentor was my partner.

One particular call weekend I received a call from a very good friend with whom I had trained in residency. He was now president of the medical staff at the hospital where we had trained. I'll never forget that conversation; I know it word for word. He told me The Mentor had been killed in a private plane crash a couple of hours before. I had dealt with unexpected and traumatic death throughout my seven years as an emergency room physician—but nothing like this.

All of a sudden, I didn't want to do medicine anymore. I wanted to throw away my pager, walk out of that hospital, and never look back. I had to find a place to be alone, and it was a few hours before I could compose myself to even get through the day. I didn't sleep at all that night, thinking about The Mentor and that I would never see him again. I had thought he would always be around. I would cry, then lie there and think about all that we had been through; sometimes the tears would break into a smile, as I thought about some of the funny things, only to have my eyes well up over and over. I got through the weekend, but only because I knew that he would not have had it any other way.

I could not bring myself to attend his memorial service. I know I should have, and I'm sure he's pissed at me for not attending. I called another partner and talked to him about it and let him know I meant no disrespect, but I just couldn't go. Maybe I felt a part of me had died, too, and I just couldn't fathom that. I am not certain I am any closer to resolution.

The Mentor has been gone for a while now. I think about him often, and it still causes my eyes to fill with tears. Sometimes I catch myself trying to take a shortcut in patient care or an examination and I feel him … he stays with me all the time. Much of who I am as a doctor is because of him, and he taught me a work ethic as a clinical scientist. He affected many people this way.

As I continue to reflect, I remember the worst call weekend ever in my life, when I lost The Mentor. I have come to the conclusion that there were very much three tragedies that day: The Mentor died and medicine lost one of its very best physicians, but more than that, I had never told The Mentor that I loved him and what he meant to me. And that is my never-ending tragedy.

Post Hoc

I have little to add to this. My mentor was Karl R. Brinker, M.D., C.M., F.A.C.P., F.R.C.P. (C). I shared this story a while back with his wife, Mary. She shared some things with me I will always hold near to my heart, and they made me miss him all the more.

I also shared this story with a few of my colleagues and friends at Dallas Nephrology Associates. I so much appreciated the time each of them took to write me a note of thanks or to share their thoughts or tell another story about Karl.

Karl has been gone for a few years now, but I still find myself hearing his voice or laughing. I've dreamed about him many times since his passing. When presented with a particular clinical dilemma, I still ask myself what I think Karl might have done in this same circumstance.

Like everyone who knew him, physician and patient

alike, I am a better person and a better doctor because of Karl. I could never repay him for all he did. I do not know if people who have left this life can "see" us or know what it is we go through, but sometimes I wonder if Karl looks over my shoulder or prompts me to do something that just might keep me out of trouble.

So, Karl, if you can hear me, THANKS!!! I love you like my family.

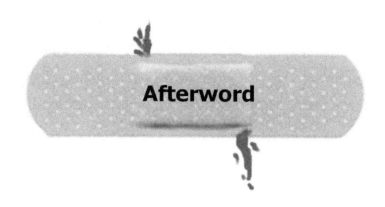

Afterword

I never cease to be amazed at the wonder of medicine. I have always been enamored with the science and the practice, going back to my formative years in grade school. I would go with my mother to the public library and check out books related to surgery and medical science. I even did a science project on anatomy and used the old Raquel Welch poster from *One Million Years B.C.* as my anatomic model—what a specimen. I'm not sure my teacher appreciated it, but I know the guys in my class did. I never missed an episode of Medical Center with Chad Everett as Dr. Joe Gannon, or *Marcus Welby, M.D.*, with Robert Young and James Brolin. In later years I became a fan of *Ben Casey* reruns. While I was pondering a career in medicine, I watched every episode of *St Elsewhere* … couldn't get enough of it. But you know what? They never said anything about call nights on those shows. I mean, really, to be real you need call nights in there somewhere.

I really do not know if I ascribe to the theory of "things happen for a reason," or we are all predestined to this or that by fate. I sometimes think things just happen. For the religious-minded person, that is not a contradiction to the theory that all things work together for good; it just means that things happen without necessarily any rhyme or reason. How they work together is how they work together.

I do know that certain personality types gravitate to certain types of jobs and that mine seems suited to medicine. I cannot stand to be second best at anything I do, and I hate to lose—pretty good traits to find in someone who is fighting for your life.

So, having said all of that … while there are some days I could walk away from medicine and never see another patient, I know, like a bad habit, I would be back. In that way maybe I was always supposed to be a physician. At times, I feel I got lost along the way and now I'm here.

As I look back on all of the call nights I have survived, some bring me to absolute belly-laughter and some bring me to tears. Sometimes I get too close to my patients; it can be wonderful to know them, but so hard when you lose them. And I have lost more than a few of my friends on call nights. I have kept vigil with family members while taking care of my patients. For some, I have orchestrated his or her exit from this life. For others, I have even carried their coffin to the grave for those who've asked me … more than a few in my years.

Wonderful and terrible things happen on call nights. It all comes with the territory. The sum total of all these experiences you have read about have made me a better doctor, but more than that, a better person. And while I have learned much about medicine, I continue to learn more about myself and people.

Be kind to your old doctor; he or she will take care of you. And if you get sick at night, go ahead and pick up the phone or go to the hospital. One of us is always on call.

Post Hoc

I would only add this, and it is for new doctors, doctors in training, or anyone who wants to become a doctor. There is so much more to being a doctor than going to medical school, completing an internship and residency, and hanging a shingle to proclaim to all that you are, in fact, one of the chosen few, privileged enough to be called "Doctor." I wish I could impart to all of you what I think it means, but I can only tell you what it means to me; *you* must find out what it means to you.

I will leave you with these recommendations:

Respect all human life. As bad as you think a person's life is, remember that a bad decision here and there and many of us would be right there. Every life needs to be guarded.

Fight for those who cannot fight for themselves.

Remain humble, honor your teachers, and respect yourself.

And ... never stop learning.

About The Author

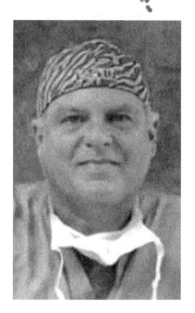

Dr. Kyle Smith (D.O., Ph.D., F.A.C.P.) is the Medical Director of Vascular Access Center Southwest Louisiana, Lafayette and a Staff Physician at the Vascular Access Centers of New Orleans, LA, North Shore, LA. and Houston, TX. He is a Consulting Physician at Our Lady of Lourdes Hospital and LTAC of Acadiana in Lafayette, LA. He was a partner with the Dallas Nephrology Associates before taking on his current duties. Smith also was an Emergency Room Staff Physician for 7 years before specializing in Nephrology (Kidney Function). His first book ER Confessional was a witty and poignant look at patients in the ER and his experiences during those years. His new release Call Nights is one doctor's journey through residency, fellowship, and private practice, along with a tribute to the Mentor that helped him become a better doctor and a better human being. He grew up in Dallas, TX, is the father of four children and enjoys hunting and fishing.

CPSIA information can be obtained
at www.ICGtesting.com
Printed in the USA
LVHW081610270119
605414LV00028B/428/P